Research Methods in Primary Care

Research Methods in Primary Care

Edited by
Yvonne Carter

Professor
Department of General Practice and Primary Care
St Bartholomew's and The Royal London
School of Medicine and Dentistry

Cathryn Thomas

Senior Lecturer
Department of General Practice
The University of Birmingham

Foreword by
Sir Michael Drury

Radcliffe Medical Press
Oxford and New York

© 1997 Yvonne Carter and Cathryn Thomas

Radcliffe Medical Press Ltd
18 Marcham Road, Abingdon, Oxon OX14 1AA, UK

Radcliffe Medical Press, Inc.
141 Fifth Avenue, New York, NY 10010, USA

British Library Cataloguing in Publication Data

A catalogue record for this book is available from the British Library.

ISBN 1 85775 198 1

Library of Congress Cataloging-in-Publication Data is available.

Typeset by AMA Graphics Ltd, Preston
Printed and bound in Great Britain by Biddles Ltd, Guildford and King's Lynn

Contents

Foreword

Two major new foci of medical care in the mid 1990s have been the strategy for making the national health service primary care led and the requirement for treatment and management to be based on good sound evidence. These two features have to be complementary, for without the latter the former has little chance of providing a base for establishing appropriate strategies or for meeting the requirements of patients. The provision of reliable data about the effectiveness of interventions in primary care has become an urgent requirement.

Research in, and into, primary care has burgeoned during the last five years. Some of this has been due to the dedication and motivation of gifted individuals, but more has resulted from the increasing influence of well-staffed Departments of General Practice. However, there are still yawning gaps in our knowledge about even some of the most commonplace activities.

There are considerable problems facing the would-be researcher in this field. Some are logistical, such as the shortage of time, space and money to support research; others are due to the fact that there is not normally a rung on the career ladder of workers in primary care labelled 'research', and so many entrants may only have the most superficial understanding of research methodology. Without this, not only is their ability to do research hampered but, more importantly, their ability to assess the findings upon which care is based is made more difficult.

For these reasons this book is both timely and necessary. More teaching of the undergraduate is taking place in primary care. It is important for the student to see that the care in which they participate is evidence based. It is important for them to understand how that evidence is collected and evaluated, and to understand that it will be their task to continue in this activity during their working lives. Registrars and new entrants to practice have the same requirements – often more pressing at this stage – and need also to recognize the pleasure and intellectual satisfaction that lies within this area of work.

Professor Carter and Dr Thomas are particularly well placed to guide the reader. Both are experienced researchers and both have track records of teaching this subject. Perhaps more importantly, they are very experienced in day-to-day clinical care, so this is not a product of an ivory tower. They have gathered together an impressive array of contributors and the result is, I believe, a book which will soon become one of the standard and well-thumbed volumes for anyone seeking to base their primary care work on a good scientific foundation.

Michael Drury
September 1996

Preface

'Good research, thoughtfully planned and carefully carried out, is one of the most compelling and absorbing of the many professional activities open to the general practitioner.'

This statement was made 15 years ago by John Howie, in his introduction to *Research in General Practice*, and although unique opportunities for research are provided in primary care, much of this research is still done by those from other disciplines. Over 90% of contact between doctors and patients takes place in general practice, but historically, general practitioners and primary health care teams have regarded research as a minority option. Family doctors and primary care nurses (practice and district nurses, midwives, health visitors and community psychiatric nurses) are in an ideal position to create a critical mass of research activity and to bid for specific funding for primary care-based research.

The medical undergraduate curriculum is going through a period of substantial change. In the past, medical students had little specific teaching on research methodology. The General Medical Council has recognized the importance of a more problem-based curriculum to equip tomorrow's doctors with a range of skills relevant to their future needs. Basic research skills are needed to permit good quality project work, when the student has an opportunity to ask a research question for the first time. As students spend more of their time in a community-based setting, more of their research will be based in primary care.

This book introduces the reader to the basic range of research skills in primary care, and will appeal to those from a wide range of backgrounds. Essentially a 'primer', it is intended to provide a solid basis for starting research in primary care and a stimulus to further exploration of the topic. Suggestions for further reading are given at the end of each chapter.

For students and established primary health care professionals, research in primary care presents an exciting opportunity. *Research Methods in Primary Care* conveys the excitement and enthusiasm each contributor feels for their subject, and will provide practical guidance for those undertaking their own research.

Yvonne Carter
Cathryn Thomas
September 1996

List of contributors

Professor Richard Hobbs
Head of Department
Department of General Practice
The University of Birmingham
The Medical School
Edgbaston
Birmingham
B15 2TT

Dr Colin Bradley
Senior Lecturer
Department of General Practice
The University of Birmingham
The Medical School
Edgbaston
Birmingham
B15 2TT

Professor Yvonne Carter
Head of Department
Department of General Practice &
   Primary Care
St Bartholomew's & Royal London
School of Medicine & Dentistry
2nd Floor
New Science Block
Charterhouse Square
London
EC1M 6BQ

Liz Ross
Lecturer and Researcher
Department of Social Policy and Social
   Work
The University of Birmingham
Edgbaston
Birmingham
B15 2TT

Dr Cathryn Thomas
Senior Lecturer
Department of General Practice
The University of Birmingham
The Medical School
Edgbaston
Birmingham
B15 2TT

Dr Sheila Greenfield
Lecturer
Department of General Practice
The University of Birmingham
The Medical School
Edgbaston
Birmingham
B15 2TT

John Skelton
Senior Lecturer
Department of General Practice
The University of Birmingham
The Medical School
Edgbaston
Birmingham
B15 2TT

Dawood Dassu
Research Associate
Department of General Practice
The University of Birmingham
The Medical School
Edgbaston
Birmingham
B15 2TT

Sue Wilson
Research Fellow
Department of General Practice
The University of Birmingham
The Medical School
Edgbaston
Birmingham
B15 2TT

Dr Martin Kendall
Reader
Department of Medicine
The University of Birmingham
The Medical School
Edgbaston
Birmingham
B15 2TT

Joyce Kenkre
Research Fellow
Department of General Practice
The University of Birmingham
The Medical School
Edgbaston
Birmingham
B15 2TT

Dr Tim Lancaster
Senior Research Fellow
Department of Public Health & Primary
 Care
University of Oxford
Radcliffe Infirmary
Woodstock Road
Oxford
OX2 6HE

Dr Andy Wearn
Lecturer
Department of General Practice
The University of Birmingham
The Medical School
Edgbaston
Birmingham
B15 2TT

David Rogers
Medical Librarian
Burton Graduate Medical Centre
Burton Hospital
Belvedere Road
Burton-on-Trent
DE13 0RB

Dr Michael Bannon
Consultant Paediatrician
Paediatric Department
Northwick Park Hospital
Watford Road
Harrow
HA1 3UJ

Dr Martin Wilkinson
Lecturer
Department of General Practice
The University of Birmingham
The Medical School
Edgbaston
Birmingham
B15 2TT

1

Why do research in primary care?

Richard Hobbs

Research on questions relevant to primary care practice, and within primary care settings, is an essential component of the overall clinical research effort. Clinical research, as a whole, encompasses a huge volume of activity within the health services of most developed countries. For instance, in the UK the Director of Research and Development (R&D) has a target to spend 1.5% of total NHS expenditure upon clinical research. In 1996 this would translate to around £700 million of NHS costs. Many authorities consider that this 1.5% target has already been reached, and indeed has probably been exceeded for many years. However, the complications of disentangling the various elements that comprise NHS expenditure make a clear statement on total research volume difficult. In addition to the indirect NHS expenditure on clinical research, the research councils and medical charities contribute around £0.5 billion per year to support clinical research. Even these sums are dwarfed by the expenditure on research by pharmaceutical and biotechnology companies in developing new products. In 1994 this figure was £1.8 billion, or 19% of all R&D expenditure by UK businesses (Anon, HMSO 1996).

The scale of the role of general practice in this huge research effort is in odd contrast with its role to service commitments in the NHS. Whereas over 90% of all NHS contacts occur and end in general practice, only a minority of the clinical research effort is either planned by general practice or takes place within it. There are many reasons for this, relating to individual practitioner issues such as the lack of availability of research training within primary care; practice structural issues such as the lack of space and time in most surgeries; major organizational issues such as the underdevelopment of academic centres of general practice; and funding issues, because so much of clinical research focuses upon molecular or specialist clinical (namely biomedical) research.

However, times are changing. Indeed, it is a symptom of the increased opportunity and optimism for general practice-based research that promotes wider publication of primary care research books such as this. The new optimism for research within general practice has resulted partially from a raised awareness of the importance of research more focused to the needs of the NHS. The consequences are that it is becoming ever more possible to perform research within primary care settings.

HISTORY OF GENERAL PRACTICE RESEARCH

Despite some of the barriers to general practitioners performing research, there is a very rich tradition of research from within the discipline. Such research tended to be characterized as being driven by individual practitioners, who were often testing their research interests upon their catchment population. Such an epidemiological approach has resulted in GP researchers making many original contributions to our understanding of the origins, scale and importance of disease.

In the 18th century Jenner conducted experiments that identified the aetiology of smallpox (Louden 1986), and thereby contributed to its ultimate eradication. Further epidemiological research was conducted in the 19th century by another general practitioner, Finlay, who observed that yellow fever was transmitted by the mosquito (Porterfield 1986). Budd (1989) performed similar research into the causes of typhoid fever and, later on in the 19th century, MacKenzie (1916) researched the epidemiology of heart disease. MacKenzie, who practised in a disadvantaged area of Burnley, also developed research interests of an applied nature, ultimately inventing the polygraph, which was the origin of the electrocardiograph.

In the early 20th century the study of practice populations was continued by William Pickles, providing rich data on the morbidity and mortality of a defined community (Pickles 1939). Pickles also went on to identify the spread of infection in infectious hepatitis. This rich tradition of a lifetime's clinical service being complimented by a long-term research interest into the epidemiology of disease within the community remains a very rich stimulus to practitioners, with more modern champions such as John Fry and Julian Tudor-Hart (Fry and Horder 1994; Tudor-Hart 1991).

Alongside an interest in the epidemiology of disease has been a tradition of qualitative research (Murphy and Mattson 1992), for example into that bedrock of clinical general practice, the consultation and doctor–patient communication. Consultation research initially focused on observations of communication, and attempted to find some explanation for the processes within a formalized structure to the consultation. This led to general practice researchers working more closely with social scientists and anthropologists. The advantage of such multidisciplinary research will often be a broadening of the focus of research. For example, in recent years consultation research has focused more upon the components of the consultation that might be used to alter patient consulting behaviour (Stott and Davis 1979). Research focus has therefore moved from research that observes what occurs, through research that raises questions (hypotheses) about the influences of these processes, to research that tests those hypotheses.

This distinction between research by lone practitioners and research by teams is important. From the examples already made, it is clearly possible for very important research to emerge from the interests and enthusiasm of individual practitioners. However, complementary research opportunities are created by a team approach, which will open up questions that an individual doctor will find difficult to answer.

Returning to the theme of epidemiology, an excellent example of the potential for team research within primary care is provided by the decennial Morbidity Surveys in Primary Care (McCormick *et al* 1995). These surveys, which have occurred in the same year as the last four censuses, are coordinated by the Royal College of General Practitioners' (RCGP) Birmingham Research Unit. This centre recruits, trains and collects data from some 150 general practice sites around the country. Very importantly, the unit also provides expertise in the interpretation of the data, alongside the research collaborators in the Office of Population Censuses and Surveys. The statistics, now in their fourth edition, represent the richest database on the morbidity of primary care populations in the world. Allied to this major decennial review, a similar network of general practitioners contributes to the weekly returns service, again coordinated through the RCGP Birmingham Research Unit (Ross and Fleming 1994).

A similar RCGP unit established in Manchester pioneered the conduct of very large multicentre general practice therapeutic trials. During the 1960s and 1970s this unit collected data on 46 000 women in 1400 general practices over a four-year period, and thereby created the largest database on the safety of oral contraception in the world (RCGP 1974). It is also worth noting that all of the data collected in the Medical Research Council (MRC) Treatment of Hypertension Trial took place within the MRC GP Framework. This study, which was the largest ever conducted by the MRC, would not have been possible without the active involvement of the participating practices.

It may appear slightly invidious to select examples of notable past GP research and researchers, but these are only described to illustrate the long history of important research that has emanated from general practice, to provide examples of some of the areas of research that have been conducted, and to contrast the potential for research of an individual practitioner with that of an active participant in a wider research team.

Where general practice has lagged behind our specialist academic colleagues is in the systematic incorporation of research into everyday practice, and the lack of substantial infrastructure to support the development of such research efforts.

WHY PERFORM RESEARCH?

There are many factors that drive research. Maintaining an interest in our clinical practice will cause us to question why the things we observe occur, and whether if we did things differently our care would improve. Being enthusiastic about one's practice therefore has a rather odd duality: enthusiasm will encourage the generation of questions to which answers can be sought, and the very process of pursuing ideas can result in enhanced enthusiasm for practice. If for no other reason, this positive feedback into enthusiasm for practice is a good reason to perform research.

This would have been a very important driving factor for some of the pioneer researchers who developed interests from long-term – often lifelong – interaction with their patients. It is not surprising, therefore, that the questions these doctors researched had direct relevance for their patients, in terms of the origins and potential treatments of serious illnesses.

The fact that so much GP research is patient specific is another very good reason for encouraging more research in primary care. Researching better ways of providing care to patients with diabetes can have immediately demonstrable benefits to those patients (always assuming that the package of care test produces positive results). Research into the genetic basis of diabetes may have crucial significance for the health of future generations of diabetics. However, there may well be a very long lag phase between such research evidence and implementable findings. Health service research, such as the evaluation of diabetic care models, is highly complementary to research programmes on more molecular aspects of the disease.

Perhaps one of the deficiencies of clinical research to date has been the almost exclusive emphasis upon biomedical research at the expense of more applied research questions. It is therefore a happy coincidence that a refocusing of the needs of the health service towards a primary care-led NHS have been mirrored by development of health services research priorities within the national NHS R&D Programme. The interest of such programmes will often relate more closely to the sorts of questions that might emerge from investigators in primary care settings. So, a further good reason for performing research in primary care is that it is becoming somewhat easier to obtain support for such research.

There are many clinical areas which have a high relevance for research interests in general practice. Research into the epidemiology of health and illness within community-based populations remains important, for example to provide estimates of disease occurrence (incidence) and long-term impact (prevalence) on the less selected populations served in general practice, rather than the highly selected populations in hospitals. There also continue to be opportunities to explore questions on the origins of disease, be they acute clusters of illness (such as the identification by a local GP of river chemical pollution at Camelford) or the prediction of influenza epidemics.

Epidemiological research relates to questions about the health of populations served by general practice. As was discussed earlier, a further research area of high relevance to our discipline relates to questions at an individual patient level, for example the expanding interest in behavioural change models and the potential for lifestyle modification at an individual level. Pursuing questions of this nature has stimulated a greater interest in qualitative research methods, and thereby facilitated closer links with social science researchers.

For many general practitioners their interest in a more academic approach to practice comes from their involvement in teaching. General practitioners have long taken a lead in the seriousness and effort they put into teaching at postgraduate – and indeed undergraduate – levels. Interest in teaching creates many secondary opportunities to perform education research, be it the evaluation of teaching pro- grammes or questionnaires on perceived educational needs. The recent interest in evidence-based medicine has created opportunities to bridge educational research with clinical research in terms of the evaluation of implementation programmes for clinical guidelines. This area of research falls squarely within the development component of R&D, and will become even more important as a mechanism for reducing the increasingly unacceptable variation in standards that operates at practice level. It is difficult enough to develop clinical guidelines based on good evidence of effectiveness; it is even more difficult to develop methods of ensuring that the guidelines that are generated are actually adopted in practice. In view of the volume of health care provided in general practice, such implementation research is of great relevance to researchers in the community (Haines and Jones 1994).

It is difficult for clinical generalists to imagine any area of condition-led research which does not have relevance for general practice. Many questions about the com- mon conditions we treat remain unanswered. There is therefore an ongoing stimulus to perform research which helps answer common and basic management decisions, such as: Is physiotherapy of any benefit for patients presenting with chronic or acute backache? Are there clinical or cost benefits associated with *Helicobacter pylori* eradication in patients with non-ulcer dyspepsia? Does the availability of open- access contraceptive clinics, or advertising the availability of hormonal emergency contraception, reduce the unwanted pregnancy rate? The difficulty for many novice researchers in primary care is not the generation of ideas for research, but rather focusing on answerable questions. The objective of a book such as this, and the increasing opportunities for research methods training, are to assist the new or less experienced researcher to develop a mechanism to progress research ideas.

OPPORTUNITIES FOR RESEARCH IN PRIMARY CARE

Despite the rich traditions of research in general practice, the multiple stimuli to performing research and the wide opportunities for study, there remain many barriers to undertaking such research. Many of these are covered in the various sections of this book. One can start by observing how to frame research ideas or to consider the methods that might be used, by regularly reading from the widening range of research publications publishing primary care studies. Peer-reviewed research-based journals are an extremely useful source of ideas. Such information is available at local postgraduate centres if personal subscription is not an option.

Many more opportunities currently exist for attendance on short courses in research methods, and even residential seminars for doctors and nurses with a more substantial interest in research. There are now a number of taught Master's courses in the UK on subjects such as primary care, public health, evidence-based medicine and health services research. For both doctors and nurses, structured support is built into research-based higher degrees, such as Masters or PhDs (Williams 1990), based on the staff in undergraduate and postgraduate departments. MDs are a further research higher degree, but suffer the difficulties of being unsupervised, resulting in there being limited support for conducting the research.

Prolonged study leave is a sensible way of building in protected time for research adopted by a limited but increasing number of general practitioners. Enhanced opportunities for clinical research fellowships are a further new and welcome option for novice researchers. Such posts are often based within undergraduate departments of general practice and funded through national bodies such as the Medical Research Council, Wellcome Trust, RCGP, or university departments themselves. The RCGP has also recently experimented with funding the infrastructure to support research at a practice level (Gray 1996). Such attempts to support additional staff time and space are likely to become more widespread.

In summary, the relevance of research in primary care has never been greater. Many very important questions remain to be answered. Individual enthusiasm, the ability to seek advice and attention to detail, coupled with a well-framed question and access to support where needed, should go a long way towards converting research interests into ongoing projects.

Further reading

Anonymous (1996) *Forward Look at Government Funded SET.* HMSO, London

Louden I (1986) *Medical Care and the General Practitioner 1750–1850.* Clarendon Press, Oxford.

Porterfield JS (1989) Yellow fever in West Africa: a retrospective glance. *BMJ.* **299**: 155–7.

Budd W (1873) *Typhoid Fever.* Longman's Green, London.

MacKenzie J (1916) *The Principles of Diagnosis and Treatment in Heart Infections.* Hodder and Stoughton, London.

Pickles W (1939) *Epidemiology in Country Practice.* John Wright, Bristol.

Fry J and Horder JP (1994) *Primary Care in 12 Countries: a comparison.* Nuffield Provincial Hospitals Trust, London.

Hart JT (1991) The inverse care law. *Lancet.* **1**: 405–12.

Murphy E and Mattson B (1992) Qualitative research and family practice: a marriage made in heaven? *Family Practice.* **9**: 85–91.

Stott NC and Davis RH (1979) The exceptional potential in each primary care consultation. *Journal of the Royal College of General Practitioners.* **29**: 201–5.

McCormick A, Fleming D and Charlton J (RCGP, OPCS, DHSS) (1995) *Morbidity Statistics from Primary Care. Fourth National Study 1991–92.* HMSO, London.

Ross AM and Fleming DM (1994) Incidence of allergic rhinitis in general practice, 1981–92. *BMJ.* **308**: 897–900.

RCGP (1974) *Oral Contraceptives and Health.* Pitman Medical, London.

Haines A and Jones R (1994) Implementing findings of research. *BMJ.* **308**: 1488–92.

Williams WO (1990) A survey of doctorates by thesis among general practitioners in the British Isles from 1973 to 1988. *British Journal of General Practice.* **40**: 491–4.

Gray DP (1996) Research primary care practices. *British Journal of General Practice.* **45(399)**: 516–17.

2

How to identify a research question and get started

Colin Bradley

IDENTIFYING THE RESEARCH QUESTION

Research has been described as 'organized curiosity', and certainly research should be driven by curiosity. Thus, the starting point for all research is a question in the mind of the researcher. However, not all questions are amenable to research, and anyone wanting to do research will need to identify from among the many questions arising out of curiosity those that are suitable. Questions that are not in a form suitable for research may need to be transformed into a research question first. However, given that *relevant* research questions are more likely to arise from practical experience of doing the job, I would suggest that as a first step you write down all the questions that come into your head about your work: carry around a little notebook or piece of paper with you for a day or two and make a note of any questions that strike you. If what arouses your curiosity are not questions as such, but rather puzzling observations, note these instead. Another way of generating questions is to brainstorm, either alone or with others, to produce the questions that most need answers. These ideas and observations can be turned into questions and categorized later into those more suitable and less suitable for research. It is important to tackle things this way round, because if one begins by thinking of a question that fits the model of a 'research question' one may end up doing research that answers research questions but bears little relationship to the actual work of looking after patients. This is a constant risk for people working in a research environment, but it ought to be actively avoided by those who have more freedom of choice. By beginning with questions arising in the course of one's work one can be more confident of producing an answer with some clinical relevance. If the question has to be modified into a form suitable for research, one can at least recall its connection with a real clinical situation, whereas research derived purely from the answers to other research questions runs the risk of becoming increasingly irrelevant. Furthermore, questions that appear initially to be unsuitable for research will often have buried within them a researchable question.

Box 2.1 Identifying the research question
- Jot down any questions that come into your head about your work
- Keep a note of questions or puzzling observations as you go about your work
- Brainstorm questions about your work (ideally with others)
- Start with practical questions and turn them into research questions later, not the other way round

---

QUESTIONS NOT SUITABLE FOR RESEARCH

The kinds of questions that are not usually amenable to research include straightforward questions of clinical diagnosis (such as 'Has this patient got angina?'); metaphysical questions (such as 'Does God exist?'); unethical questions (such as 'Would saline injections encourage or discourage "heartsink" patients from attending so often?'); questions where the answer is already very well known (such as 'Do inhaled steroids help people with asthma?'); questions that are too specific or particular to a single situation (such as 'Why does Mrs Smith come every week when there's nothing the matter with her?'); questions that are too large or general to be answerable within the compass of a single project (such as 'Does health promotion work?'); and questions that are purely definitional (such as 'Does anaemia result from a reduced haemoglobin?'). Table 2.1 gives further examples of questions generated in a day's work, with an indication of their research potential. Even among these, only metaphysical questions, unethical questions and questions of definition are precluded from research by conventional means. Things that are supposedly known beyond dispute may still be wrong. For instance, it is commonly supposed that children with vomiting and diarrhoea should not be given food, but recent evidence indicates that this may not be true. Failure to question the prevailing wisdom might have resulted in this study never having been done. Highly situation-specific questions may often be reframed into research questions. Thus the question of why Mrs Smith comes every week when there's nothing wrong can be reframed into a question about why any patient comes to the doctor when they have no

Table 2.1 A sample of questions collected by the author in the course of one day's work in an inner city general practice

Original question	Suitable for research?	Reason	Comments
Are home visits worthwhile?	No	Too broad	What proportion of home visits are medically essential? Might be more researchable but more work on definitions etc. required
Why do some people with asthma still smoke?	Yes		Would need some exploration of the size of the problem and will probably need a qualitative approach
Is this lady's rash eczema or tinea coporis?	No	Clinical diagnosis question	Answered by normal procedures of clinical diagnosis
What is the best treatment for chlamydia?	Yes	Appears to be a simple clinical question but is amenable to research	Research required is most probably secondary (literature-based) research
Why are Friday evening surgeries such a pain?	No	The answer is fairly obvious on one level, and it is a bit metaphysical on another	There is probably a human psychology thesis in this, but its not a question for primary care research in my opinion!
Do single mothers consult more often than mothers in a stable relationship?	No/Yes	Answer already known (but perhaps not well enough known/established)	This has been done but has not been well publicized. The answer, interestingly, is 'No'. The determining factor is probably an effect of deprivation
Why does Mrs Hunt not leave her violent husband?	No	Too specific	The research question is probably more to do with why women remain in violent relationships (on which there is existing literature); there are primary care questions about how we detect and manage problems of domestic violence

Table 2.1 *continued*

Original question	Suitable for research?	Reason	Comments
Is paranoia in an alcoholic man due to his alcoholism or is it a manifestation of schizophrenia?	No	To an extent this is a clinical question and to an extent it is a question of definitions	There are several research questions that could be generated around co-existence of mental health symptoms/problems in single patients
How safe is hydrocortisone 1% cream in infantile eczema?	No	Answer largely known although the evidence on long-term use may be unreliable. Further research, however, may be unethical	There may be several research questions within this that are answerable such as 'are GPs prescribing hydrocortisone 1% for infants and if so how much, what for, with what results etc.?'

obvious illness. Large questions can be broken down into smaller ones. Thus a project looking at whether or not giving people advice about exercise results in a change in their behaviour will cast some light on the question of whether or not health promotion 'works'. What more often leads to the failure of research to produce useful results is not so much the lack of a suitable research question, but rather a disorganized or poorly focused curiosity which has not generated a proper question at all. Examples of this abound. One hears the perpetrators describing their research in terms such as, 'I am just looking into the role of the GP in health promotion', or 'I am doing research on patients' consulting behaviour'. Such imprecise language often betrays vagueness of thinking and lack of rigour in the approach to research. Indeed, what such woolly thinkers often do is take a perfectly good question and turn it into something much less incisive. The moral is, once you have got your question keep it clearly in mind, as it is all too easy to drift into the quagmire of 'looking into' things with no clear purpose.

Box 2.2 Questions not suitable for research
- Questions of clinical diagnosis
- Metaphysical questions
- Unethical questions
- Questions to which the answer is already well known
- Questions that are too situation specific
- Questions that are too large or broad
- Questions of definition only

WHAT MAKES A GOOD RESEARCH QUESTION?

Professor John Howie, in his seminal book on, *Research in General Practice* (see Further reading), provided simple, clear guidance on what makes a good research question. He identified a good research question as being one which is important, interesting and answerable. Importance may derive from the commonness or severity of the medical condition being investigated, or from the possible implications of the answers to the question. The importance of a question can be gauged by thinking through how policy or practice might be altered if the research produces its anticipated results. Thus the test of importance is 'Will the results change anything of any significance?' If it is difficult to visualize much changing even if the research answers the question it sets out to address, one has to wonder whether the research is worth doing. What makes a research question interesting is even more difficult to determine, but again there is an acid test: tell a few people you are hoping to do some research to answer your question and see how they react. If you are consistently greeted with a lack of enthusiasm you might question the value of your proposed research, or you might need to ask whether you have tested it on the right people. Answerability is also relative, and depends on the extent to which one has or can acquire research methods that might allow the question to be answered. This is very difficult for a novice researcher to gauge, as questions that seem easy and straightforward may look fraught with difficulties to a more experienced researcher, whereas questions that may seem to defy a research approach may be much more susceptible to research than you might have supposed, because of the availability of a methodology or approach of which you were unaware. Therefore, in assessing the answerability of your project seek advice from as many expert sources as you can. Answerability is also dependent on resources. Thus if your time or access to investigational material or other resources are limited your question may be unanswerable by you, but this is not to say that it is unanswerable per se. The ultimate evidence of answerability is, of course, successful completion of the research project.

Box 2.3 Features of a good research question
- Important
- Interesting
- Answerable

HYPOTHESIS OR QUESTION?

Some purists would insist that research should start not with a question but with a hypothesis. At its most simple, a hypothesis is a testable idea arising from one or more observations. This idea is subjected to various tests involving the collection of further observations, with or without an intervention having taken place. The basic research question is, therefore, 'Is this hypothesis correct or not?' Although not all research questions worthy of exploration will necessarily fit into this straitjacket, it is often worth trying to see if your research idea can be framed as a hypothesis, or whether your own starting point has been such a hypothesis or hunch. If the research question does not actually address an existing hypothesis (yours or some-one else's) then it is probably setting out to generate new hypotheses. If that is so, you should consider whether what you are going to get is the answer to a qualitative or a quantitative question. Consider, too, whether it might not be possible to collect data within your project which might shed some light on the truth or otherwise of hypotheses so generated. To give an example from my own work: I began with a question of whether or not the prescribing of new drugs by hospital doctors was a major factor in the subsequent uptake and prescribing of these drugs by general practitioners. Stated as a hypothesis this would be that hospital doctors' prescribing of new drugs is not a major influence on the prescribing of general practitioners (the convention is to state the hypothesis in its negative form, the null hypothesis, i.e. what would be true if the hypothesis fails the tests?). One might, of course, have no initial hypothesis, and so the research question might have been 'What are the major factors that influence general practitioners in their prescribing of new drugs?' With this more general question one can still anticipate that the hypothesis about the influence of hospital doctors might emerge, and so one might, while studying the influences on GPs of new drug prescribing, collect data on the prescribing of hospital doctors, so that one could subsequently be in a position to test hypotheses about this aspect. Whether your research is setting out to test one or more hypothe-ses, or is more likely to generate hypotheses for subsequent testing, it is essential that before embarking on any other work you must clarify the aims for the research and, ideally, write them down.

GETTING STARTED

Having devised your hypothesis or identified your research question, there is a very strong urge to dive in and get on with it, but this must be resisted. Many research projects fail because the researcher has rushed headlong into the question without considering all the possible pitfalls. The key to good research is careful planning. Even well-planned research sometimes goes wrong, but poorly planned research nearly always goes wrong. Planning a research project involves several steps, not all of which have to be gone through in every instance, but all of which should be considered. The first step consists of checking that the research question is indeed a good one and worthy of your time and energy, and your or someone else's (if you are lucky) money. The question should be subjected, several times ideally, to the tests of importance, interest and answerability suggested above. This will involve talking to other people, but be careful about how, when and with whom you do this. You should probably not expose your research idea to the scrutiny of others too early in your thinking about it, unless you can be pretty sure a negative reaction will not put you off completely. When floating your idea for discussion do not trivialize it, making it too easy for others to reject; nor should you allow yourself to be too attached to it, so that if others criticize it you will not be demoralized. It is also important to consider to whom you should expose your idea. Although it is good to consult someone experienced in research – ideally someone doing research in the same clinical context as you (i.e. primary care) – beware of the inevitable tendency of experienced researchers to incorporate your idea with thoughts of their own, and, knowingly or unknowingly, to begin to divert you and your project into something of theirs. It is also a good idea to talk through your ideas with someone who is experienced in primary care but not in medical research. They also may have a tendency to want to divert you towards something of more interest to themselves, but with a little tact and diplomacy they can usually be confined to providing you with feedback about the worth of your proposed research. People more experienced in the field can give useful tips to ensure that the project is more successful, e.g. by giving you hints on how to recruit participants to your study.

The next decision to be made is what methods are to be employed to investigate the question. You may already have come up with ideas as to how the question could be answered, but it is important not to just launch the research with the first methodology that comes to mind. It may be that the study you thought could obviously be done using a questionnaire, should really be done by face-to-face interview; or that the study you felt could be done by collecting data from your own practice actually needs data from several practices to have any reliability. Once again, the most important thing for the novice researcher (and even the not so novice researcher) to do is to seek help and advice from others. If the study is essentially quantitative it is important to speak to a statistician, preferably a medical statistician. If it is a clinical trial speak to a person who has done clinical trials. If it is an epidemiological study speak to an epidemiologist. If the study is going to be essentially qualitative speak to an appropriate social scientist. If you are not sure whether it is qualitative or quantitative, Chapter 4 should offer some guidance, although it is still important to consult widely on your choice of methods.

Having chosen the methods, you should next think of the resources you will need to carry out the project. Resources consist mainly of time, money and physical facilities. Who is going to do the research may seem a fairly superfluous question, as the answer may seem to be that it will be you. However, this is not necessarily the case: it is usually wise to get some help with the research, or at least elements of it. Many aspects of data gathering and handling can very competently be handled by ancillary or secretarial staff in a practice. As it is not part of their basic job description it may have to be paid separately, but it will often still be worth it as their time may be cheaper than yours and they may be more keyboard proficient, for instance. It may also be worth considering employing or deploying other staff on your research, as this gives you a strong incentive to seek funding (Chapter 3). Having your project funded brings additional benefits, as it obliges you to do the project and to an agreed timetable, which often imposes a useful degree of discipline. It also involves subjecting the project to some form of external scrutiny, which can give further insights into the proposal's importance, interest and researchability, and referees will often provide useful hints or pointers as to how the project might be improved (whether or not they eventually agree to fund it). Deciding how much money to apply for is a skill in itself, and once again you should seek expert advice from experienced researchers. The question of physical facilities may not arise if the study is to be done in your own practice, although the implications for the practice premises should be thought through. If the research is being done outside your own practice, consent from others is needed to use their facilities, in addition to other consent required for ethical reasons.

The benefits of doing a pilot study cannot be recommended too highly. If, for instance, you hope to do a project which compares two ways of providing treatment in a group of patients, you should pilot all aspects of the study. This would include piloting how one might recruit doctors and/or patients to the study; piloting any data-collecting equipment, which might include case report forms, questionnaires or interviews; and piloting any analytical techniques you plan to use. For qualitative studies, too, doing some pilot work is also essential. Two other important points about pilot studies need to be borne in mind. First, you need to be aware of the possible effects of contamination of your study by the experience gained by research subjects in the pilot. Therefore, wherever possible the pilot work should be done in a different population or area from the main work. Secondly, you should be prepared to undertake more than one pilot study, especially if you are new to research. This is because pilot studies can sometimes show up fatal flaws in the research design, leading to such a dramatically different project design that the new methods need to be piloted before the main study commences.

Having warned you against rushing in, it behoves me to warn you against endless procrastination too. Once you have your idea and have talked to lots of people for advice, it is important you do not then sit on it. Get out and do some pilot work. Once you start on this the feeling of doing something and generating results will, hopefully, give your project the next vital boost to its momentum.

Box 2.4 Key steps to getting started with a research project
- Think of a practical, clinically relevant question
- Convert the question to a researchable question if necessary
- Check that the question is suitable for research: test for importance, interest and answerability
- Decide on methods to address the question
- Ascertain and try to obtain the resources needed to complete the project
- Seek ethical and any other approval required
- Conduct one or more pilot studies
- Avoid rushing in, but also avoid endless procrastination

Further reading

Armstrong D and Grace J (1994) *Research Methods and Audit in General Practice.* Oxford University Press, Oxford.

Howie JGR (1989) *Research in General Practice* (2nd edn). Chapman & Hall, London.

McNeil P (1985) *Research Methods.* Routledge, London. (Now available in a second edition, published as part of the 'Society Now' series.)

3

Writing a research proposal and getting funded

Yvonne Carter

WHY WRITE A RESEARCH PROPOSAL?

There can be no doubt that unique opportunities for research are provided in primary care. Many GPs, practice and community nurses want to undertake research, but are unsure how to proceed. For any research you do, even the smallest and most humble studies, it is wise to prepare a statement about what you intend to do and how. This is more formally known as a **research proposal** or **protocol**. Producing a research proposal requires careful preparation, as it helps to formulate the whole plan of the study, putting it into perspective with regard to time, cost and outcomes. This chapter outlines the stages involved in writing a research proposal. For a simple study it need be no longer than one or two pages, but several drafts will normally be needed. For a relatively straightforward study, such as establishing your consultation rate over one week, it may seem that even this effort is unnecessary. However, writing a research proposal is a good habit to start and you will discover that even with an uncomplicated study there will be times when a plan is invaluable.

The process of research starts with asking questions and ends with publishing results. The process of writing a research proposal will provide both a clear plan of action and a framework for the final report. Writing the proposal will in itself require time, thought and patience. Many people find it difficult to express their ideas clearly in words, and may find that they are impractical anyway, when written on paper. Putting ideas on paper before you start a project can be very useful in identifying problems with the research: it enables you to assess whether you have an answerable question and a viable method, and makes you condense your thoughts. Show your proposal to other colleagues and ask them if it seems coherent and reasonable. Don't forget to listen to their comments and advice: most projects set out with overambitious questions or hypotheses. Discussion with colleagues and peers is very important in working up any research proposal. Prepare the groundwork well and you will save time later. The final version will provide the stimulus for the paper you eventually hope to publish!

WRITING A RESEARCH PROPOSAL

There is no uniform format for a research proposal. The length will vary according to the type of research approach planned and the size, duration and complexity of the study. The type of information contained within the proposal will, however, remain more or less the same. Some funding agencies produce their own standardized forms, e.g. the National Research and Development Programme has its own two-page application form for outline proposals, and guidance notes on completing the form are provided. If shortlisted, a much more detailed submission will be necessary and the application form may be provided on disk.

In general, to ensure that nothing is omitted the researcher can use the following steps as a checklist (Table 3.1). The proposal has a **Project title**, a **Summary**, a **Background** to the study, a statement of the **Aims and objectives**, a description of the **Methodology** you have chosen to use, a **Timetable** for the project, the **Funding** requirements or **Costings**, and finally the **References** used to illustrate the background. Increasingly research proposals submitted for funding must also include a discussion of the **Generalizability** of any recommendations from the study, a description of the **Benefits** that the proposed investigation will bring to the NHS, and a description of how the research findings will be **Implemented**.

Table 3.1 Eight steps in writing a research proposal

1 Give yourself a working project title
2 Summarize the project
3 Give the background to the study, with appropriate references
4 Decide on the aims and objectives of the study, or formulate a hypothesis
5 Briefly describe the methods to be used, including design of the study, ethical considerations, data collection and analysis, interpretation of results, report writing and potential benefits to the NHS
6 Describe the project milestones and devise a timetable to enable you to check that all stages will be covered and time allowed for writing up
7 Describe the likely costings for the project
8 Apply for funding, if required

Project title

The proposal must have a title, sufficient to tell any funding body or the local research ethics committee what the project is about. You will only be ready to devise a final title when you are clear about the focus of the study. Try to show that you have planned the study with an open mind, for example 'A study to determine whether . . .'. It is usually necessary to give your name and an address for correspondence after the title.

Summary

The summary is an important part of the proposal, as it must impress the reader and encourage him/her to read on. It needs to be brief but explicit, and usually no more than 200 words are required. Although the summary acts as an introduction or overview to the study, it is easier to write after the whole proposal has been completed and the exact plan of action is clearer in the researcher's mind.

Background

This section sets the scene, gives the recent history of the topic and summarizes the relevant literature. Avoid including a huge list of references within the proposal: it is better to concentrate on a few that are particularly relevant. The review of the literature should demonstrate knowledge of previous research, how the project relates to it and how it will add to it. It is important to read enough to enable you to decide whether you are on the right lines. The initial reading may also give you ideas about the approach and methods to choose. The background will assert the importance of the chosen topic and state its professional relevance. Previous research should be competently described and appraised, and any deficiencies highlighted. The purpose of the study and why it is appropriate to be attempting it at this time need to be stated.

If appropriate, describe the expertise and prior knowledge contained within your research team. It is especially important to highlight why you are ideally placed to carry out the proposed research, e.g. a successful pilot study, adequate patient numbers, facilities in place, previous experience of carrying out a health technology assessment. A short curriculum vitae of each applicant is usually required. Large bids for funding are more likely to be successful if there is a demonstrable mixture of skills and professional backgrounds in the applicants.

The aims of the project should then follow in a logical step from the background.

Aims and objectives

The question or hypothesis must be clearly stated in this section of the proposal. The aims are the overall **goals** of the project, and the objectives are the **specific tasks** in a stepwise sequence which will lead to the goal. The aims and objectives should be listed in order of importance. They should be shown to be manageable within the study's timescale and budget. It is therefore necessary to think carefully about what is and what is not worth investigating.

Research methodology

A plan of the investigation, including the research methodology, follows. It is at this point that you are expected to describe the proposed work and give an outline timetable. Funding bodies and local research ethics committees will pay particular attention to this part of the proposal.

Specific details of the overall study design are described, i.e. what, how, where and when it will be done, and you must adequately justify why the chosen experimental design is suitable. There is usually no need at this stage to include particular instruments, such as questionnaires. It is only necessary to outline what form of data collection you are planning to carry out, e.g. the rationale for choosing self-administered questionnaires as opposed to structured interviews or focus groups. Details of the population to be involved, the sampling technique to be used and the actual numbers must be provided, e.g. all asthmatic patients attending the practice asthma clinic over a six-month period, estimated from historical records to be 120 patients. It is sensible to acknowledge and address where there may be difficulties, e.g. anticipated response rate or recruitment of patients. If established protocols are available, refer to these where possible.

It is important to define what you mean by a 'case' for the purpose of your study, how you plan to ascertain your cases, and whether you are using controls. If you plan to use a case control study a power calculation should be included, stating the projected sample size. This will be covered in more detail later in the book. What you describe in the methods section should be referred back to the objectives, to ensure that the information being collected is sufficient and that you are resisting the temptation to collect data which are unlikely to be relevant.

Details of the method are followed by a brief overview of what you intend to do in the **analysis**. For an ambitious project it is advisable to consult a statistician early in the planning stage. Unless your project is a purely descriptive study, you will need to indicate how you are planning to compare measurements or outcomes between groups, for example the use of a standard database and statistical package.

Timetable

Devise a simple timetable to enable you to check that all stages will be covered and that time is allowed for writing up. Give the proposed duration in months, and identify anticipated stages/milestones (Figures 3.1 and 3.2). In general, research time can be divided into thirds, one-third for planning and getting ready, one-third for data collection and one-third for data analysis and writing up. It is easy to take too

		Time (weeks, months)					
		1	2	3	4	5	6
Start project							
Tasks:	1	*	*				
	2		*	*	*		
	3			*	*		
	4			*	*	*	*
Finish project							

Figure 3.1 A simple Gantt chart.

long over one stage and so to have insufficient time to carry out essential tasks in the next. Most researchers particularly underestimate how long it will take to write up a project. Consider also whether it is possible to set aside some protected time each week, during which you can escape from clinical and administrative responsibilities. If you can, you should!

Generalizability, benefits to the NHS and implementation of research findings

For a small study it is not usually necessary to include a discussion under these headings. However, for applications to the National R&D Programme it is usually a prerequisite. A discussion of the generalizability of the research findings to primary care as a whole will depend on the proposed setting and method of sampling. For example, a study to investigate the knowledge and attitudes of patients or staff about asthma from a large rural fundholding practice may be completely different from those in a single-handed inner city practice. You will also need to explain how the proposed study will address the specified R&D need (usually only one area), giving the potential benefits to the NHS in terms of health gain and/or cost reductions or efficiency gains. Dissemination and implementation of research findings is in itself a huge topic, but may include presentation at scientific meetings (local, national and international), conferences and workshops, and publication in peer-reviewed journals, reports and newsletters.

Funding requirements or costings

Justification of the financial support needed requires some thought before submitting an application for funding. Even for quite a small-scale study the printing and mail-

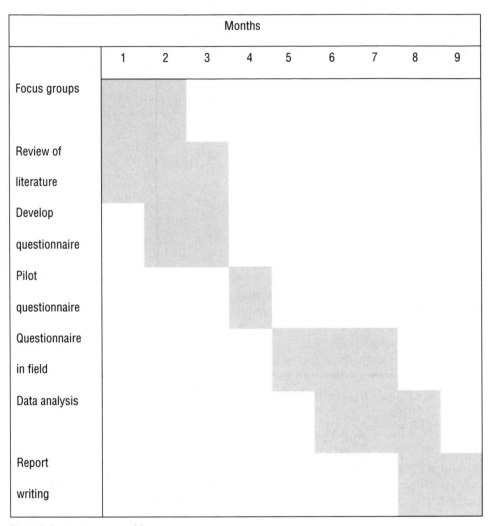

Figure 3.2 Project timetable.

ing of a questionnaire can be expensive. You will need to prepare costings so as to get an overview of your funding requirements. Costings divide into three main sections: labour, equipment and consumables and miscellaneous, e.g. travel expenses. All these should be carefully itemized even if you hope to fund the project from petty cash. For employed staff outline staff numbers, grades and timescales, with a breakdown of national insurance and superannuation contributions. Grant-giving bodies, in particular, will expect the costs to be realistic. Financial arrangements will be simplified if projects start on the first of a month.

The NHS wants to see more research being done in primary care, which means that individual members of the primary health care team should have a better chance of getting funding than ever before. General practitioners and members of their teams are in an ideal position to address the health needs of their patients, to create a critical mass of research activity and to bid for specific funding for general practice-based research.

When applying for funding it is obviously essential to decide how much money you need. It is also important to decide whether you are going to do the research on your own, with other members of your practice team, with other colleagues, or as part of an academic unit. If you are applying from a university, for example, a member of the finance department will need to check and sign your application before you send it, and will usually add indirect staff costs (commonly 40% over-heads) and VAT, where applicable, to the final amount.

Each region has a regional director of R&D, an R&D manager and support staff. The regional R&D directorates manage nationally and regionally funded R&D programmes. National priority programmes of R&D managed by regions on behalf of the Central Research and Development Committee include cancer, mental health, cardiovascular disease and stroke, the primary/secondary interface, physical and complex disabilities, and mother and child health. These topics are obviously relevant and important to primary care-based researchers.

Increasingly, regional R&D directorates are developing initiatives in primary care and are planning to facilitate the involvement of primary health care teams in research work, not just in clinical studies but also in evaluating different methods of delivering health care. Increasing numbers of research facilitators are being ap-pointed to give advice on an individual or practice basis. In some regions assistance in preparing a bid is available. Those interested in applying for funding should contact their local R&D department for details and an application form. The remit is usually wide and cases are considered on their merits. All bids have to go before a committee, which includes representatives from general practice and local health authorities.

Many regions are also appointing 'research general practices', where funding is given to support the infrastructure costs of doing research rather than supporting an individual project. This initiative has followed the example of the research practices supported by the Royal College of General Practitioners (RCGP). The RCGP has also funded a number of research training fellowships in recent years, to provide protected time for practice-based research, to promote a research culture in general practice, and to encourage higher degrees. Historically, the Scientific Foundation Board of the RCGP has also been active in supporting general practice-based research. The College maintains a useful database of grant-giving bodies, with details of the timing for applications, the upper financial limit and specific topic areas.

Research monies for medical and clinical audit are also becoming more widely available. Your local Medical Audit Advisory Group (MAAG) or health authority would be a good point of contact for identifying such funds. Money from Trust funds is sometimes set aside particularly to promote research activity for specific pro-fessional groups, e.g. the Claire Wand Fund of the British Medical Association and the Rudolph Friedlaender Memorial Fund for general practitioners and the Derek

Bloor Trust for practice nurses. Consulting a local practice nurse group or the nurse facilitator/adviser at the health authority may help to locate such funding. Project funding linked to health promotion activity is often advertised in the nursing press and is worth looking out for, and occasionally travel scholarships are also available. Finally, many drug companies will make available small grants for specific subject areas.

References

References to the literature are placed at the very end of the proposal, and should be accurate and well set out. You may choose only a small number of references (fewer than ten) at this stage and list them in one of the standard styles, i.e. Harvard or Vancouver. The latter is probably the most popular style and involves numbering the references in the text, either in parentheses or superscript, in the order in which they appear. One or more references to the same article use the same number. They are then collected together at the end of the proposal.

In summary, research is not a difficult activity although it does require the ability to think clearly in an organized way. Writing your thoughts formally as a research proposal will be useful in giving you a clear idea of what its all about.

Figure 3.3 Example of research grant application (funding not included)

1. Project title
Aggression and violence in general practice: an evaluation of different models of training for members of the primary health care team.

2. Project summary and objectives
The objective of this study is to develop an appropriate model of training for members of the primary health care team in the management of aggression and violence in general practice. The cost-effectiveness of two alternative models of training (multidisciplinary education versus unidisciplinary training) and current practice will be evaluated in a three-arm randomized controlled trial. The alternative models of training are designed to make appropriate use of the skills and time of the professionals involved and to provide training which is fully centred on the needs of primary care workers. The evaluation will include an examination of indicators of productivity and effectiveness based in a primary care setting. It will focus on a comparison of the inputs, outputs, impact and outcomes associated with the different models of training.

3. Background to the project
It has long been realized that health care workers are at risk of violence in their working environment. The extent of the problem is illustrated in various reports

and in the media.[1-5] New regulations require employers to evaluate risks to staff, to assess what action needs to be taken in order to reduce this risk and to undertake the necessary remedial action.[6] One problem in tackling violence at work is a denial of its magnitude by staff and managers alike.

Not all violent episodes can be averted, but appropriate training in the prevention and management of violence can decrease the likelihood of staff injury. The applicant already has an established record of research activity in the area of aggression in general practice. The need for expertise in primary care, communication skills training, economic evaluation of health care provision and behavioural science in designing, implementing and evaluating packages of training is also reflected in the team's composition. A training pack (video and written training guide) has already been developed for members of the primary health care team to address some of the issues around violence in general practice.

4. Plan of study including research methodology

AIM The aim of this study is to evaluate alternative models of training for members of the primary health care team in the management of aggression and violence in general practice.

CONTENT OF TRAINING The package will generally raise awareness of the issues relevant to primary care, and includes various training activities. The pack is designed to encourage the setting up of practice procedures to combat and prevent aggression and violence. The focus will be on training tailored to the needs of primary care-based professionals and geared towards minimizing problems by providing information and support. The exact details of these alternative models will be developed and piloted in the development phase of the study, but the main differences from current opportunistic training will be practice-based multidisciplinary team training and training of unidisciplinary groups from a variety of practices (e.g. groups of practice managers, GPs, community nurses). The effectiveness of training will then be evaluated in the different practices.

A systematic review of the literature will also be undertaken to inform the development phase, together with detailed consultations with relevant professionals. To assist members of the team at various stages of the project, a steering group will be set up to include other experts in the field.

STUDY POPULATION Recruitment of staff for training will take place in general practices. Practices will be selected to achieve full demographic representation of staff and to represent the spectrum of practice size, location and fundholding status. Practices will be randomly allocated to an arm of the study.

DATA COLLECTION AND ANALYSIS The effectiveness of each model of training will be assessed in terms of a variety of outcome measures and the costs of each will be estimated. Self-administered piloted questionnaires will be given prior to training to relevant professionals from each practice recruited to take part in the study. At the completion of each training session each participant will be asked to complete an evaluation form. Training sessions will also be recorded and the tapes transcribed for qualitative examination by modified content analysis to determine themes.

The data on physical and psychological health of the primary health care staff and their satisfaction with training will be assessed through a postal questionnaire at six months after training. An initial sample of 50 practices will enable 15 practices to be included in each arm, assuming a dropout rate of 10%.

GENERALIZABILITY To inform the development of a national programme, the findings of the study must be generalizable in different practice settings, so a large representative sample will be required for training.

DISSEMINATION The results will be published via peer-reviewed and non-peer reviewed articles. Presentations will be given locally, nationally and internationally.

OUTLINE PROJECT TIMETABLE Anticipated starting date of project is 01/01/1997. The project is of two years' duration, to incorporate development, piloting and training; follow-up at one year; analysis and presentation of results.

Time (months)

0	3	6	9	12	15	18	21	24

Start project

Tasks: 1 ------------- (Practice recruitment)

2 --------------- (Questionnaire to staff)

3 ---------------------- (Training)

4 ---------------------- (Follow-up questionnaire)

5 ---------------------- (Analysis)

Complete project

5. References

1. Health and Safety Commission, Health Service Advisory Committee (1987). *Violence to Staff in the Health Services.* HMSO ISBN 0118839179.

2. Department of Health and Social Security (1988). *Violence to Staff; Report of the DHSS Advisory Committee on Violence to Staff.* HMSO, London.

3. Harrington JM (1990). The Health Care of Health Workers: The Ernestine Henry Lecture. *Journal of the Royal College of Physicians of London.* **24**: 3, 189–95.

4. Harris A (1989). Violence in general practice. *BMJ*. **298**: 63–4.

5. Thomas B (1995). Risky business. *Nursing Times*. **91**: 52–4.

6. Stark C, Paterson B (1994). Violence at work. *BMJ*. **308**: 62–3.

Further reading

A number of R&D publications relevant to the NHS R&D strategy are available from: Room 449, Department of Health, Richmond House, 79 Whitehall, London SW1A 2NS.

4

Qualitative vs. quantitative research methods

Colin Bradley

A DEFINITION OF QUALITATIVE RESEARCH METHODS

It is not easy to define qualitative research methods without resorting to the rather tautological assertion that they are methods that are not quantitative. The definition is as least as much about defining what the methods are for, as defining them per se. Therefore, my own definition of qualitative research methods is that they are methods for the collection, analysis and interpretation of data on phenomena that are not easily reduced to numbers or that might be destroyed by any attempt to do so. One is thus obliged to stipulate what is meant by qualitative phenomena. The example I often use is 'love'. Love is a phenomenon that is fundamentally qualitative. One can do quantitative research on various aspects of love – for example how many people say they experience it or have experienced it; what people do when they are in love; how often people admit to making love, etc. All these things could be described as research on love but they are not. They are about manifestations of love, but they are not about the thing itself, and mere counts of this or that aspect associated with love seem, if anything, to diminish rather than increase our understanding of the phenomenon. However, in-depth descriptions of individual experiences of love – such as in love stories – do enhance our understanding of the phenomenon itself. Health is another phenomenon which could be said to be fundamentally qualitative in nature.

EXAMPLES OF QUALITATIVE RESEARCH METHODS

This definition is probably best amplified with some examples. Perhaps one of the original methods that is exclusively qualitative is that of 'participant observation', and is particularly associated with the early development of anthropology as a discipline. Originally it involved the anthropologist going and living in the social world of others whom he or she sought to understand, typically in those days 'undiscovered' African tribes. By 'immersing' him- or herself in the social world of the subject tribe, the anthropologist would be able to understand the culture in greater depth than would be possible from any lesser degree of involvement. Field notes, transcripts of conversations and cultural artefacts, along with explanations of their meaning to the tribe and so forth, constituted the 'data'. The chief worry about these methods seemed to be about the possibility of the researcher 'going native', and hence losing objectivity or the ability to report fully on his or her observations – or in some instances failing to report at all. From the idea of total immersion in another social world derives the idea of research involving lesser degrees of immersion, which are usually described as 'non-participant observation'. In this type of research one seeks to obtain the same sort of understanding of other people's construction of the social world but without the immersion in their life that is implied in participant observation. In reality, observation is never either entirely participant – one can never actually go completely native – or entirely non-participant, in that to gain people's trust sufficiently to understand them one must to some degree give up one's objective stance. Thus participation or non-participation in sociological observation is never absolute, but is always just a matter of degree.

Many examples of qualitative research, including both participant and non-participant observation, will usually involve some interviews. Interviews are usually classified as structured, unstructured or semistructured. Again, this suggests a rather greater differentiation than is truly the case. There is no such thing as a totally unstructured interview, as all interviews are structured in real time by the participants, either consciously or unconsciously. Here, too, it is merely a matter of degree, with some interviews having more or less clearly defined structures or being more or less focused on one or more topics. 'Focused interview' is another term you will hear which suggests more rather than less structure.

Some other bits of jargon you will often hear bandied about in social science methodological discussion are ethnology, ethnography and ethnomethodology. These words all derive from the Greek *ethnos*, meaning nation. It is the same word that gives rise to the more commonly used word 'ethnic', referring to a supposedly culturally homogeneous group. Ethnography and ethnology are used to refer to the study of peoples and cultures (ethnography is, strictly speaking, the *description* of peoples and culture, and ethnology the actual *study* of them) and hence they overlap substantially with anthropology. Ethnomethodology is a word used to encompass some of the methods used, but is particularly associated with the American ethnographer Garfinkel, who described particular methods used to uncover the unwritten (usually subconscious) rules that govern the behaviour of people and groups of people. A much-quoted and classic example of Garfinkel's approach was his instruction to students to behave in their homes as if they were visiting guests rather than residents. The technique is an example of the 'incongruity procedure'. It can more simply be described as 'breaking the rules'. The irritation this behaviour would engender would often lead to the open and verbal expression of codes of behaviour or expectations of behaviour than were otherwise usually just accepted and understood.

Conrad Harris, Professor of General Practice in Leeds, used his Pickles lecture entitled 'Seeing sunflowers' to draw the attention of GPs to what he perceived as the lost skill of pathography. Pathography is more or less the use of detailed description of diseases in individual cases to enhance our overall understanding of people and their diseases. Pathography is really just the skill of ethnography applied to the particular context of medicine.

There is a host of other terms that describe various aspects of the qualitative research tradition. Many depend on the analysis of artefacts, usually written, such as archives, literature, reports etc. Such documentary material is analysed using techniques broadly described as 'content analysis', although this term is sometimes used more precisely to refer to specific quasistatistical approaches to such material. Other methods rely rather more on oral accounts and histories, sometimes described as 'narratives'. Other less familiar and conceptually more difficult terms include phenomenology, hermeneutics, grounded theory etc.

Box 4.1 Some examples of qualitative research methods
- Participant observation
- Non-participant observation
- Unstructured (sic) interviews
- Semistructured (sic) interviews
- Focused interviews
- Ethnology
- Ethnography
- Pathography
- Ethnomethodology
- Content analysis (some forms of)

WHAT QUALITATIVE RESEARCH METHODS ARE GOOD FOR

It is already implied that what qualitative methods do most effectively is help explain the social world and social phenomena. Although this is indeed true, there are other particular strengths to qualitative research methods that allow their application to a vary wide variety of research questions, including some that are much more practical and specifically medical, and not just descriptive. Thus, they can be used to test or examine hypotheses or models, although they are most suited to hypothesis or model generation. In medicine, for instance, such sociological models as the Health Belief Model have been derived from qualitative research, but they have also been tested using qualitative techniques. Qualitative methods are also useful for comparing the views of social groups. For instance, in order to understand the perspective of two groups such as doctors and patients on an issue – such as, say, genetic screening – the natural choice of research method would be a qualitative one. On other occasions one may wish to study social networks, or the interconnection between people in a community, for instance how different doctors influence each other in their clinical practice. This would involve qualitative research techniques, particularly those usually referred to as sociometry. Just as epidemiology can be used to assess the impact of physical agents or events on a community's health, ethnological techniques can be used to study the impact of social events, such as the introduction in 1990 of the new contract for GPs. Other chiefly sociological phenomena, such as medical pluralism (i.e. the idea that patients can simultaneously participate in allopathic medicine and other alternative techniques such homoeopathy), are almost only amenable to qualitative research techniques. Similarly, the whole phenomenon of 'deviance' (in its sociological sense) is best studied by qualitative techniques, and indeed may not be researchable by any other means. Thus the study of such phenomena as the sexual practices of prostitutes or the behaviour of the drug-taking subculture is almost impossible using any other means. Less extreme examples of 'deviance', such as drug non-adherence (non-compliance), although researchable by quantitative means, is probably best approached qualitatively if the phenomenon is to be understood rather than just documented. Finally, qualitative methods are particularly suited to understanding groups of people and their behaviour, in addition to that of individual people. Thus they can be used to understand the behaviour and needs of particular subgroups of society, such as single parents, the elderly, ethnic minorities, and even such sociologically bizarre groups as doctors!

Box 4.2 What qualitative methods are good for
- Study of explanatory models (e.g. Health Belief Model)
- Comparing different perspectives of different groups (e.g. doctors and patients)
- Identifying social networks
- Assessing the social impact of events
- Studying medical pluralism
- Study of deviance (e.g. non-compliance)
- Understanding behaviour of social groups

FEATURES OF QUALITATIVE RESEARCH

It is now worth considering which features of qualitative research methods differ from those of quantitative methods, and what features they share in common. In qualitative research methods the emphasis is on an accurate or true reflection of social reality (telling it like it really is) rather than on precision (saying how much it is like this or that). Thus, to this extent numbers are not of the essence in determining the worthiness or otherwise of a piece of research. This is often taken to mean that numbers are of no consequence whatsoever in qualitative research, but this would be overstating the case. One qualitative researcher I know of was so adamant that numbers were antiethical to qualitative research that she would not even number the pages of her research reports; this is definitely taking things to extremes. Numbers do matter, in that to understand the social world one usually (but not invariably) has to talk to more than one person and get more than one perspective. However, the numbers required to ascertain the veracity or otherwise of a contention generated by qualitative research are certainly fewer than is usually the case for quantitative research, where the strength of the argument being put is often crucially dependent on the numbers involved. Thus in qualitative research the sample size cannot often be determined in advance, in the way that it often can be in quantitative research. In many forms of qualitative research what limits the numbers required is the arrival at a point at which one seems to have 'bottomed the problem', or when additional data collection seems to reveal no new information or insight. This is clearly a matter of judgement. Sometimes the limitation on the sampling frame is one of feasibility or funding, although this less than ideal scenario sometimes applies equally to quantitative research.

Another feature of qualitative research is the nature of the end product. Data in quantitative research are clearly numeric, and can usually be condensed by the use of mathematical tools, most notably those of statistics. The conclusion can usually also be stated in the concise form of a theory or hypothesis with, ideally, some measure of the precision of that conclusion, such as a confidence interval or P value. In qualitative research the data usually take the form of verbatim quotations from research participants, often referred to as respondents or informants. Often these quotations will be organized into a framework or template, which illustrates how they support each other in reaching the conclusions. The conclusions will sometimes be expressed as a theory or hypothesis, but more often as a social construction or model of how the world is with regard to the topic of the study. This clearly presents difficulties in communicating the research results within the traditional IMRAD (introduction, methods, results and discussion) framework imposed by most scientific journals. The end product of qualitative research is also more likely to be a better or clearer description of how things are, rather than predictive of how things might be. That is to say that qualitative research is more naturalistic and descriptive than experimental, although, as mentioned above in relation to ethnomethodology, this is not an exclusive feature. Likewise, qualitative research is more likely to generate hypotheses than to be used in testing them, though again this is not an absolutely distinguishing feature. Qualitative research methods can be used to generate descriptions and hypotheses, and quantitative research methods can be used to test hypotheses.

However, it must be recognized that the nature of conclusions will still vary in terms of what the quantitative tradition refers to as reliability. Thus anything concluded from a piece of qualitative research is likely to be probabilistic rather than deterministic, and is more context specific than generalizable. From the usual standards of quantitative research these features (probabilistic and context-specific conclusions) appear to be inherent weaknesses in qualitative methods, but to think this is to fail to understand that quantitative and qualitative research yields different sorts of knowledge, and that to judge qualitative research by quantitative standards is mistaken.

This raises the important issue of how one can establish the worth of a piece of qualitative research. To consider this, one can usefully discuss the features the methods have in common. Both qualitative and quantitative methods attempt to be 'scientific', by which it is meant that they seek to produce, by an approach that strives very hard to steer clear of sources of error, an understanding of phenomena that is reasonably true and trustworthy. One of the cardinal features of both approaches is the quest for rigour in method and interpretation, and the consciousness that truth is never absolute but always open to challenge, as long as the same standards of scientific rigour are applied. In quantitative research the means to these ends are well described and, in the medical community at least, reasonably well understood. Thus one has learnt to look out for sources of bias and how these are dealt with, and one seeks evidence of reliability and validity, and both of these can, to a degree, be defined and measured. Establishing the trustworthiness of qualitative research is, to those unfamiliar with the tradition of this type of research, rather more difficult. Fortunately, though, there are corresponding measures of the trustworthiness of qualitative research and means of identifying their presence or absence (Table 4.1). Thus, corresponding to the concept of reliability there is the concept of dependability, and corresponding to the concept of validity is the concept of credibility. The means to these ends are also described, and include such techniques as triangulation (deriving data from several perspectives or sources); member checking (feeding back one's conclusions to the original respondents and checking whether they agree with you); searching for disconfirming evidence

Table 4.1 Corresponding terms describing trustworthiness of quantitative and qualitative research, and all-embracing terms relating to the rigour underpinning all research

Quantitative research	All-embracing term	Qualitative
Validity	Veracity	Credibility
Reliability	Consistency	Dependability
Objectivity	Neutrality	Conformability
Generalizability	Applicability	Transferability

(actively seeking any evidence that might refute the conclusions); and thick description (giving complete tranches of unedited data, along with information on how they were condensed, edited or categorized so that the reader can arrive at their own judgement on the links between data and the model postulated).

It is most important to understand that qualitative and quantitative research are not mutually exclusive, but are rather complementary approaches which, when used together, will usually reveal more about the world and how it works than will either used alone. This is not to contradict what has been said above about certain areas and topics more naturally lending themselves to qualitative research, and likewise certain topics lending themselves more naturally to one or other approach. The kind of knowledge produced by such different endeavours is different, but neither type is in any absolute sense superior or inferior to the other, and in the progress of medicine, as was stressed in the introduction, both types of knowledge are required.

WHY QUALITATIVE METHODS ARE PARTICULARLY SUITED TO GP RESEARCH

Despite the above comments on the value of both methods of research to the overall progress of medicine, there are some reasons why qualitative methods commend themselves particularly to GP researchers. These relate to the nature of general practice, which is more closely affiliated to the social world than the world of investigative natural science, and as 'people' we are particularly interested in people as social beings (rather than just as physiological systems) and in the meaning of social events. Qualitative research is also more holistic and less reductionist in its approach to problems which, again, fits well with how we as GPs work. The acceptability of small numbers explored in greater depth also makes these methods more feasible to GPs. I often say that GPs make poor epidemiologists (who are intrinsically quantitative in their approach), because if we see something once we are inclined to dismiss it as an insignificant rarity, but if we see it twice we are inclined to perceive it as an epidemic. This problem of seeing a little of everything but not much of anything is not such a problem in naturalistic qualitative enquiry. GPs are, indeed,

---

Box 4.3 Why qualitative methods are suited to primary care research
- Focus on people as social beings rather than as physiological systems
- Shared concern with the meaning of events for people
- Holistic approach
- Small numbers are acceptable
- Depth of understanding may be acquired over time
- Access to 'private worlds'

in the position of both non-participant and participant observers of many aspects of people's lives. We can also observe people and social worlds over long timescales in a truly anthropological style, in which the depth of understanding often increases over time rather than in proportion to the amount of data collected over a short period of time. We also have access to people's private worlds, although, as happens in cases of similar access in any qualitative research, this does bring with it certain ethical problems and constraints.

I would also argue that GPs already have some of the skills needed to become good ethnographers, although these will require some adaptation to the research task. GPs already use interviews and social and personal histories as major tools of their trade. It must be made clear that there are important differences between the research interview and the medical interview, mainly as regards the extent to which the respondent is helped and encouraged to respond to the interviewer in a way that ignores his or her status as a doctor. GPs, too, are interested in social events and the meaning of these events for people. GPs see their patients in their cultural context, in which GPs may have a special place. GPs are, or ought to be, open-minded because of their exposure to illness in the early stages, which means that we are used to unexpected findings and poorly organized data. These are all desirable attributes of an ethnographer. Therefore, it can be said with some justification that GPs are already natural ethnographers.

Box 4.4 Why the good GP is already an ethnographer
- Uses case histories as main investigative tool
- Takes a social and personal history
- Allows patients to express the meaning of events
- Sees patients in their cultural context
- Already belongs to the community under study
- Open-minded (few preconceived notions)
- Used to unorganized illness
- Open to the unexpected

Further reading

Crabtree B, Millar WL (1992) *Doing Qualitative Research*. Sage Publications, London. Number 3 in 'Research Methods for Primary Care' series.

McNeil P (1985) *Research Methods*. Routledge, London. (Now available in a second edition, published as part of the 'Society Now' series.)

Norton PG, Stewart M, Tudiver F, Bass MJ and Dunn EV (1992) *Primary Care Research: Traditional and Innovative Approaches*. Sage Publications, London. Number 1 in 'Research Methods in Primary Care' series.

5

Qualitative research methods – data collection and analysis

Liz Ross

As we learnt from the last chapter, qualitative research attempts to present the social world, and perspectives on that world, in terms of the concepts, behaviours, perceptions and accounts of the people it is about. The research methodologies used are therefore approaches that collect data which is 'raw' or natural, i.e. what people say or do in 'real' life situations. The methods of analysis are inductive in the main, in that a particular case or a small number of cases are studied in depth and then theories or generalizations to other contexts are suggested from the researcher's interpretations. Qualitative research methods are also holistic, in that both in terms of the data collected and the way the analysis is designed, the context and the various dimensions of a situation or account are included. Each aspect of the research area is viewed as part of a whole picture.

Qualitative research methods allow the researcher to work with the raw data, to explore the nature of the stories people tell or the way they behave, to look at the different perspectives, understandings and interpretations that social beings bring to each social situation in which they participate. Thus the methods used by the researcher to collect and analyse qualitative data need to allow those data to be collected and worked with in their 'natural' form. The researcher's role is to listen and observe and then interpret or make sense of what she or he sees and hears. As the extent and nature of the data cannot be known before they are collected, the processes of collecting and analysing qualitative data often intermingle. The collection of some data from perhaps a small number of in-depth interviews may be followed by analysis, which then helps the researcher to identify further data that are needed to test out or develop his or her preliminary interpretations. For example, if some research was being conducted into patients' experiences of waiting to see the doctor, initial interviews might suggest that people waiting by themselves have a different experience from those waiting with children. The researcher might then want to investigate whether the experience was different because they were waiting with another person, or whether it was specifically because they were waiting with children. Thus further interviews could be carried out with people who were waiting with other adults.

In both the collection and the analysis of qualitative data the researcher is the primary instrument, the person who hears the story, observes, reads, records and interprets. Thus the researcher is in close touch with the real situation of the data, close to the ground.

COLLECTING THE DATA

Qualitative data are often relatively unstructured: they come in the form presented by the subjects of the research, rather than being prepackaged by the researcher. The researcher needs flexibility and adaptability to respond to the research subjects, rather than imposing a structure upon them. The researcher is, in effect, creating a natural situation, be it a conversation or a group discussion, or observing a natural situation, in order to collect the data. Qualitative data come in many forms, and the ways of collecting are limited only by the researcher's imagination and skill. They include:

- Semi- or unstructured interviews, individual or group
- Stories, poems
- Diaries
- Documents, reports, minutes
- Observations of situations and events, participant or non-participant
- Videos, pictures, photographs
- Others!

The two most commonly used of these sources of qualitative data are in-depth interviews and group interviews, often called focus groups.

IN-DEPTH OR SEMISTRUCTURED INTERVIEWS

An in-depth interview is a conversation between the researcher and the subject about the research area or topic. It is designed to allow the respondent to tell their story in their own way, while ensuring that the aspects the researcher wants to explore are covered. It also allows the subject matter to be explored in some

---

Box 5.1 Characteristics of structured questionnaires and semistructured interviews

Structured questionnaire	**Semistructured interview**
Asks the same questions of each respondent using the same wording and typically has a limited range of possible answers	Allows the respondent to express their ideas in their own way using their own words and determining the range of aspects and issues they want to raise

---

depth to discover the nature of the experience, feelings and perceptions of the respondent.

Conducting an in-depth interview

An in-depth interview has a broadly defined agenda which arises from the research questions that have been identified. These provide the boundaries for the discussion as well as suggesting a structure for the conversation. An interview guide is usually prepared.

An interview guide:

- Helps the interviewer to remember the points to cover
- Suggests ways of approaching and talking about topics
- Reminds the interviewer about probes and ways of asking questions
- Includes an introduction and a way of ending the interview
- Ensures that the interviewer covers all the topics
- Gives a possible order of topics
- Helps the interviewer to enable people to talk in their own way, and as fully as possible.

A interview guide is not a list of questions but rather an aide mémoire for the researcher.

Beginning the interview

The first questions should be designed to put the respondent at ease and to help them to begin to talk. Asking them to describe their situation or something that has happened to them will help them to feel they have something to say, and will begin to give them a clearer idea of the nature of the interview.

The body of the interview

The interview then moves into the areas of particular interest to the researcher, and as the interview progresses the rapport between researcher and respondent develops and more detailed or sensitive areas may be discussed. The respondent may not talk about the topics raised in the same order or way that the researcher has anticipated, and he or she must be prepared to be flexible and to come back to explore in more depth areas that have been mentioned but not developed by the respondent.

Ending the interview

As the interview draws to its close the researcher moves on to less sensitive and more general matters. The respondent should be reminded again that the interview is confidential, and the researcher should ensure that the respondent is content with the way in which the interview has developed.

Recording the interview

In-depth interviews are usually recorded and then transcribed. Although most people are willing to be recorded, the researcher must always be prepared to make notes if they are not willing. The interviewer must be familiar with the tape recorder and have sufficient tapes and batteries. The volume and voice levels must be checked at each interview, and the tape should be checked immediately after the interview while the event is still memorable. If notes are being made these can be limited to reminders during the interview and then written up as fully as possible immediately after the event, using the interview guide as a reminder of the areas covered.

FOCUS GROUPS

A focus group is:

- A group discussion
- Focused on a particular topic
- Has members who have something in common
- Led by a facilitator
- Time limited
- Task limited.

Focus groups are used as a research method to find out what groups of people think and how they discuss issues and ideas together. Most people form their opinions and attitudes from both their own experiences and their awareness and discussion of other people's experiences and ideas. The focus group therefore attempts to recreate a natural phenomenon: a group of people with something in common discussing an issue, an experience or an event. A focus group is not used to find out what each individual thinks or has experienced, but rather how the *group* discusses the topic being researched. The group will often be given a task. The group discussion is then

> **Box 5.2 Tips on in-depth interviewing**
> - Remember the interview is a conversation, not an interrogation
> - Have a naive curiosity: don't assume that you understand what the respondent means – ask:
>   'Can you tell me more about that?'
>   'Can you tell me how you feel about that?'
>   'In what way was that a good/bad experience?'
> - Try to sit at an angle to the respondent and maintain eye contact
> - Don't be thrown if they say something which shocks or surprises you
> - Look expectant, nod encouragingly, say 'That's interesting!'
> - Use probes to encourage people to tell you more:
>   'What happened next?'
>   'Can you tell me more about . . .?'
>   'You said earlier that . . . can we talk a bit more about that?'
>   'How do you mean?'
>   'In what way?'
> - Embarrassing situations and sensitive issues may be tackled by:
>   'What about you? How do you feel about that?'
>   'Some people say that . . . what do you think about it?'
> - Avoid double questions, e.g. 'How do you feel about going there with other people and having to do what they want to do?'
> - Avoid leading questions, e.g. 'Don't you think it would be better if . . .?'
> - Don't sum up what people say: rather, say:
>   'Am I right in thinking that you . . .?'
> - Don't interrupt the flow if they don't immediately answer the question, but don't let them stray too far away from the topic – gently bring them back!:
>   'That's very interesting; I wonder if we could now move on to talk about . . .?'

structured to allow the group to discuss the issues before moving on to complete the task, which may be, for example, to identify the most important points that have been raised in the discussion, or to prioritize areas for improvement in service provision.

Running focus groups

Like the in-depth interview, the focus group has a beginning, a middle and an end.

- *Beginning* – getting people talking, relating experiences and ideas.
- *Middle* – helping people to focus by asking more specific questions.
- *End* – completing the group task.

The focus group facilitator prepares a guide to help in structuring the discussion while allowing the interaction between the members of the group to develop. In the example given below, the participants are first all asked to say something about themselves and then are asked to discuss a number of different aspects of visiting their family doctor. Questions are directed to the group rather than individuals, and the facilitator's role is to generate discussion rather than lead a question-and-answer session. Each section ends with a focus question to help the participants to reflect on the discussion. Towards the end of the discussion the group is asked to complete the task of identifying the improvements people would most like to see.

In setting up a focus group consideration must be given to how many people to invite and whether they should or should not know each other. A group discussion usually works well with between eight and 13 participants. More should be invited, as it is likely that some will not attend. Focus groups can work equally well with established groups as with people who have not met. The venue and the time should be arranged to facilitate the particular group, and some thought should be given to offering incentives for people to attend. If possible, the facilitator should be assisted by a co-facilitator, who can ensure that practicalities such as the arranging of chairs, the welcoming of latecomers and so on do not distract the facilitator from his or her role of facilitating the group discussion.

Tips on running a focus group discussion

- If a person is not taking part try to draw them in by asking if they have anything to add. Try to remember something they have said so that you can do this at an appropriate time.
- If one person is dominating the discussion, it is acceptable to say politely:
  'Thank you for that; now I think we need to hear what other people think'
- If two or more people are talking at once, deal with it immediately:
  'Can . . . make her point first and then . . . please?'
- If two or more people are having their own conversation, deal with it at once:
  'Do you want to say something to the group?'
- If two or more people are arguing about something and excluding others, step in with:
  'There are clearly different points of view on this; can I just check . . . feels this way . . . and . . . feels that way . . .? What do other people think?'
- Do not assume that you understand what someone is saying; encourage people to say more and to explain or describe their point, using phrases like:
  'Can you tell us a bit more about that . . .?'
  'How did you feel when that happened?'
  'Is this something that other people feel/have experienced?'

Note these phrases on the topic guide so that you can remind yourself if necessary.

Box 5.3 Focus group guide – going to the family doctor/GP

Thank you for coming along; this will take about an hour, and anything you say here will be confidential in that none of you will be identified in any report about the meeting. We are doing some research to find out what people think about going to see their family doctor and we are particularly interested in any ideas you may have about how this service could be improved.

I'd like to start by asking each of you to introduce yourself by just saying your name and saying about how long you have been going to your current GP.

1. **How did you first decide to go to that particular surgery or health centre?**
    ⇒ Other members of family – did you consider going elsewhere?
    ⇒ Change from other doctor – why did you change?
    ⇒ What did you think would be the advantages of your choice?
    > Do you think people have enough information about GPs and health centres?

2. Can we think now about going along to see the doctor? Some doctors' surgeries have an appointment system: **what do you think are the good points about having an appointment system?**
    ⇒ In what way is that good? Can you tell us a bit more about that?
    ⇒ Any other good points?
    And what are the difficulties about having an appointment system?
    ⇒ In what way is that difficult?
    ⇒ Any other difficulties?
    > How do you think the system could be improved?

3. Sometimes you will have to wait before going in to see the doctor: **how do you feel when you have to wait?**
    ⇒ What sort of thing makes the waiting better?
    ⇒ What makes it worse?
    ⇒ Should some people get in to see the doctor more quickly than others?
    > What is the maximum time you think people should have to wait?

4. In some health centres and GP surgeries you can now also see other people like nurses, social workers and chiropodists, as well as go to various special clinics.
    Do you have any information about the other people and services at your surgery or health centre?
    ⇒ How did you find out about those services?
    ⇒ What are the advantages of having other services there?
    ⇒ What are the disadvantages?
    > How do you think people can be kept informed about the health services in their area?

5. **What improvements do you think people would most like to see at their GP's surgery or health centre?** (List on flipchart and discuss priority ranking)

ANALYSING QUALITATIVE DATA

Objectives of analysis

Unlike the analysis of quantitative data, qualitative data analysis is not dependent on quantifying and looking for statistical relationships. Rather, the researcher is the primary analysis instrument and is concerned with making sense of and interpreting the data collected. During the analysis the researcher seeks to uncover and make visible the experiences and perceptions of the research subjects by exploring the data for:

- *Conceptual definitions*: how people perceive situations, other people, ideas
- *Typologies*: classifications or groupings of people or situations that tend to have common characteristics, opinions and experiences
- *Associations*: ideas and experiences which are often associated with particular situations or people
- *Explanations*: why something happens in a particular way
- *Illumination*: data that 'shed light'.

Methods

There are various approaches to the analysis of qualitative data, but all have three key characteristics:

1. The approach must be rigorous and systematic. Raw qualitative data can be extensive and varied, and organizing the material so that it is easy to work with is essential if the researcher is not to drown in paper. The data should be worked on systematically, so that the same analytical processes are applied to each section. The process of analysis itself should be recorded so that the researcher's thinking and approach can be visible to others.

2. The analysis focuses on the raw or grounded data. The researcher works with the raw data rather than transforming them into codes or numbers, thus keeping in touch with the data well into the analysis process.

3. The analysis is a dynamic process. It is not decided and laid out beforehand, but develops through data collection, reflection and analysis.

Stages of analysis

Although there are different techniques used to analyse qualitative data, including the use of computer software, most approaches have four stages:

- Familiarization: getting to know the data

- Indexing: identifying parts of the data as interesting and creating an index, as found in a textbook, so that each data segment can easily be found
- Grouping data: searching for and grouping together on a chart, diagram, large sheet of paper or card index all the data segments, from each of the data sources, about a particular area of interest, so that they can be studied together
- Development of themes: working with the data to explore and test out themes and interpretations.

Completing the picture

Analysing qualitative data can be like doing a jigsaw puzzle when you have been told that it is a country scene but you have not seen the picture itself. As you first begin to sort the pieces into edges and pieces of distinguishable colour, you begin to get some clues about the sort of picture it might be. As you piece a section together you may find it is similar to, but not quite, what you thought it was, or it may prove to be something quite different. Some of the blue pieces do make the sky, but other blue pieces may be part of a boat or a door. You may also find that some pieces are missing and you have to look further to find them, although you have some idea of their shape and colour from the surrounding pieces. As you complete the edge you become aware of the boundaries of the picture and the broad areas of colour and detail. You then are able to seek out particular pieces to try, turning them around to see if they fit, rejecting them and searching for others if they are the wrong shape, but knowing that they probably fit somewhere else. When the picture is complete you are able both to see the intricacies of the picture and the whole, and to put the picture into a general category, to say this is a mountainous country scene, or a country cottage, or a lake, and compare it with other similar pictures. Remember, however, that the picture was always there: it had to be broken down into pieces to allow you to really work on it and come to appreciate both its detail and its wholeness.

Further reading

Bryman A and Burgess RG (eds) (1994) *Analysing Qualitative Data*. Routledge, London.

Kelle U (ed) (1995) *Computer-Aided Qualitative Data Analysis*. Sage, London.

Kitzinger J (1995) Introducing focus groups. *BMJ*. **311**: 299–302.

Qualitative Health Research (1995) **5**(4) (Special issue on focus groups).

Rubin H and Rubin I (1995) *Qualitative Interviewing: The Art of Hearing Data*. Sage, London.

Silverman D (1993) *Interpreting Qualitative Data: Methods for Analysing Talk, Text and Interaction*. Sage, London.

6

Questionnaire design

*Cathryn Thomas, Sheila Greenfield and
Yvonne Carter*

WHY USE A QUESTIONNAIRE?

Questionnaires are one of the most common approaches to research in primary care. They have many uses, including screening, audit and consumer satisfaction, as well as their more familiar role in research. For many of us the arrival of another questionnaire on our desk is accompanied by a significant downswing in our emotional state. Much of the reason for this feeling is that many questionnaires are not well designed. The use of the questionnaire is not an 'easy' method of research if it is done properly. To use this approach well requires a great deal of thought and piloting: do not fall into the common trap of thinking 'well, we need to do something quickly, let's do a questionnaire'.

Questionnaires are used to measure the characteristics, opinions and attitudes of the respondents to whom they are sent. Depending on the type and size of the survey, we can then hope to be able to make some general statements from the information provided which are applicable to the population as a whole. Of course, this means that we must be sure we are sampling as representative a group of the population we are interested in as possible (see Chapter 8).

Questionnaires are a useful and quick method of obtaining straightforward data from large numbers of people, but less good at finding out what one person believes in depth, in which case an interview would be better. Questionnaires can be used to find out about people's thoughts and beliefs if they include open questions, although the information will never be as detailed and in-depth as one could obtain from an interview. For many researchers the decision as regards interviewing or using a self-administered questionnaire depends not so much on the number of people one wants to sample, but on financial and time constraints. Do not be lulled into a false sense of security about the cheapness of questionnaire research, as by the time the questionnaire has been constructed, piloted, printed and distributed and reminder letters have been sent, the cost soon mounts up.

However, questionnaires, provided they are well designed, can be extremely valuable research tools, and this chapter will help you to design your questionnaire to be as effective as possible.

SITUATIONS IN WHICH QUESTIONNAIRES CAN BE USED

Self-completion by respondents

These can be either sent by post or distributed for completion in a given location (e.g. surgery waiting room), and consist of a standardized set of questions with a fixed range of responses.

Some advantages:

- Can cover a wider section of the population in a shorter time than interviewing
- Respondents complete in their own time
- Questions are standardized and cannot be altered or rephrased
- Relative anonymity: respondents do not have to speak to an interviewer and thus be personally linked to their responses.

Some disadvantages:

- May have a lower response rate than interviews as they lack the personal touch, and if people are not interested in the topic they may not respond at all
- Questions must be clear, concise and to the point, so that respondents can understand and cannot misunderstand or misinterpret them
- It is not certain whether the questionnaire has been completed by the intended respondent or by someone else.

Face-to-face interview

Questionnaires can still be structured with a standardized set of questions and responses, but are more likely to be semistructured with more of a bias towards open questions.

Some advantages:

- Tend to have a higher response rate owing to the presence of the interviewer
- They are more in-depth and detailed, and the interviewer can prompt and expand
- The interview can be tape-recorded, so that no information is missed
- The interviewer can make notes about the timing, location and context of the interview, the way in which the respondent answered the questions, and his or her manner, e.g. embarrassment, anger.

Some disadvantages:

- More costly and time-consuming than self-completed questionnaires
- The interviewer can alter or rephrase the questions depending on the situation
- If there is more than one interviewer care must be taken to ensure that interviews are carried out in a uniform way.

Telephone surveys

Some advantages:

- Convenience
- Cheaper than face-to-face interviews
- Response rates may be higher than postal questionnaires owing to the 'immediacy' of the approach; respondents have less time to think about whether they will participate.

Some disadvantages:

- The subscribers listed in telephone directories may be a biased population in terms of gender and social class
- It may be difficult to contact your intended respondent, as anyone may answer the telephone
- People may be called away from the telephone, resulting in an incomplete questionnaire and missing data.

PLANNING YOUR QUESTIONNAIRE

By the time you have decided to use a questionnaire you will obviously have thought carefully about the subject matter you are interested in, and should by this stage have a good idea of the questions you want answers to. The first step is to use the literature to find out whether there is already a validated questionnaire on your topic of interest. There are a variety of health measurement scales on a wide range of subjects. There is therefore no point in devoting a huge amount of effort into constructing your own instrument, which will not have been rigorously tested, if there is already a good questionnaire validated by previous research. It is quite legitimate, if you wish, to use questions from existing questionnaires provided they are acknowledged. Three books which are extremely helpful in this regard are *Measuring Health* and *Measuring Disease* by Ann Bowling and *Measures of Need and Outcome for Primary Care* by Wilkin, Hallam and Doggett (see Further reading).

The first thing to do when composing a questionnaire is to think very carefully about what you want to know. It is easy to fall into the trap of asking questions which interest you but are not central to the research question because you feel the 'while I am here' desire to ask about other topics as well. Keep your questionnaire as brief and clear as possible, in order to induce as many people as you can to answer it.

Try to visualize how the final results will look. It is helpful to construct draft tables to check that the necessary data are being collected. When planning to use a questionnaire it seems funny to begin at the end, but it is very useful. Make a list of the variables you intend to include in your analysis before you begin, e.g. age, sex, social class, ethnicity, deprivation score. If you are planning to compare your results with those described in other studies, you must decide whether to use identical questions or to adapt a questionnaire that has already been developed and validated for a similar situation.

It is at this stage that you are often forced really to refine your research idea. This is a good thing, and you should not feel anxious if you are forced to make decisions between certain questions. The questionnaire quickly acts as a focus for your research. Start by writing down the questions that you want answers to, then look through and see whether there are any that are extraneous to your needs. If so, strike them out and avoid the temptation to fit them in again later.

Try to draw on the experience of other colleagues, as well as your own clinical observations and knowledge of the literature relevant to your project. Each item should be related to the study objectives. This stage allows the list of variables to be elaborated, e.g. level of deprivation may be assessed in terms of living alone, renting accommodation, car ownership. For this example you may wish to include specific variables from either the Townsend or Jarman indices. The Townsend score is a measure of material deprivation and uses four variables from Census data. The Jarman index (underprivileged area score) is concerned with the increased workload for general practitioners working in deprived areas and uses eight variables.

It is best to have a mix of closed and open questions. Whereas closed questions are useful for obtaining a lot of information, subjects have no opportunity to give any spontaneous answers and cannot explain why they answer in a particular way. Open questions allow subjects to give their own answers, many of which you would not have thought of, and these are of considerable use in gaining an understanding of what people believe. Open questions are more difficult to code or categorize, but you do obtain more varied information from them.

PILOTS

Piloting the questionnaire is vital: it is probably the most important stage of all. It involves sending out a small number of questionnaires to a group of people similar to your final sample – 10 or 20 people is adequate. You will be testing the questions, their wording and format, the sequence, transition statements (e.g. the next four questions ask about . . .) and skip questions. From the responses you can also judge the clarity of the instructions in your covering letter, and the layout and length of the questionnaire (if no one finishes it you can assume it is either too long or is offensive!).

- Ask for comments and any questions you didn't think of
- Is it measuring what you intended?
- Is the wording understood, and is that understanding similar for all respondents?
- Closed questions: is there a box for all responses (people often add 'don't know')
- Are any questions missed systematically or frequently, or are they consistently answered wrongly?

From this information change your questionnaire and, if you can, repilot it.

QUESTIONS

There are four broad areas one can enquire about:

- Attributes: what people are
- Behaviour: what people do
- Attitudes: people's way of reacting to or regarding a situation
- Beliefs: what people think is true.

Questionnaires are good for obtaining information about attributes and some behaviours (bearing in mind that people will answer what they think you want to know), but not so good for attitudes and beliefs. For the latter two interviews are better, and although you may obtain some information from questionnaires it may be open to criticism.

Format

The format of the questions will depend on how the questionnaire will be administered, e.g. by telephone, by post, by direct interview, and whether the data are quantitative, qualitative or a mixture of the two.

Closed

Closed questions limit the respondents to a number of mutually exclusive responses, e.g. *Yes, No* and *Don't know*. The response 'Don't know' may sometimes be appropriate, but try to avoid the middle of the road option. Closed questions may also take the form of alternative statements, a checklist or a rating scale. The Likert scale is a popular means of recording an opinion, whereby the respondent is given a statement and is asked to tick one of the categories, e.g. A hot lemon drink will ease a sore throat: *strongly agree, agree, no opinion, disagree, strongly disagree*. The choice of a question or scale will also depend on whether the variable being measured can be expressed categorically, e.g. sex, or continuously, e.g. emotion.

In general, analysing the results is easier when using the closed answer system. However, closed questions do limit the amount of information: you get what you ask for and nothing more.

Open

For qualitative research, open rather than closed questions may be more appropriate. Open-ended questions allow the respondents to comment in their own words. The results of this format take into consideration everyone's views, but can be difficult to read and to analyse. Open questions can be useful in a pilot phase to establish the categories to be used in closed questions.

It is good practice to use a closed question before an open one: the closed question can be used for any statistical analysis, whereas the open system can be used to gauge respondents' views and opinions. The respondent should be given specific instructions when they can give more than one answer to a question, e.g. 'which *one* of the following statements is true . . .?'. Do not forget to make it clear at the beginning of the questionnaire whether you would like the respondent to circle, tick or cross the responses to your questions.

Wording questions

The wording of your questions will influence the way in which they are answered, and therefore this requires a great deal of thought. At this stage it is valuable to obtain the opinion of other people, as one of the problems with any type of question is that the asker tends to know exactly what they mean but the person being asked may well not understand. By asking the opinions of friends and colleagues you will get useful information that will help you reword the questions; you may need to do this several times. This is the prepilot stage.

Particular problems to look out for are ambiguous or imprecise questions, or those that make assumptions about the respondent's life. For example, a question such as:

> How much time do you devote to sport?
> a great deal/a certain amount/none

is ambiguous because no time frame is given. Is the answer meant to be in terms of each day, each week, each month etc.? It also assumes that the respondent knows what you mean by sport: to some people snooker may be a sport, whereas to others it is not. If you are interested in asking about physical exercise you need to be precise about what you mean, and if you are asking about time or any other variable you need to give strict parameters.

Try to avoid questions that involve the respondent having to remember incidents that are far in the past. The more obliging will reply to these questions, but the answers cannot be relied upon. Few of us can remember things that happened in the past unless they were of major importance to us, and even then our memories are not entirely reliable.

It is very easy to ask two questions in one, and when you come to analyse the results to realize that you cannot decide whether a respondent who has been asked 'do you take aspirin and paracetamol' is in fact responding 'yes' to aspirin or 'yes' to paracetamol, or 'yes' to both.

It is easy to assume that lay respondents will have knowledge that we as health professionals have. They may well not, and it is invaluable to have your question-naires scrutinized by people who are as much like your respondents as possible. This is the value of a pilot.

It is all too easy to lead people to the answer you want them to give: try and ask the question in as neutral a form as possible.

Confine yourself to asking people about things they know about, rather than things they might be able to imagine. Questions concerning how they would feel in certain hypothetical situations do not give terribly helpful answers: it is better to ask about situations that they have actually experienced.

Questions about issues that are likely to be sensitive or may offend respondents, e.g. 'have you ever had a sexually transmitted disease?' are especially difficult to design. However, you may want to know about areas that some people find difficult to talk about, and a self-administered questionnaire means that they have the option to put the questionnaire in their bin or to fill it in privately and anonymously. A variety of strategies can be used.

Instead of asking people whether or not they participate in a particular form of behaviour, one strategy is to assume that they do and then ask about it. You should include a 'never' category, so that they can deny that they do this. By giving the impression that the behaviour is acceptable the intention is that they will not feel embarrassed at admitting that they do undertake it. For example:

> How often in the last month have you had unsafe sex?
> 10–20 times/5–9 times/1–4 times/never

This is a better strategy than asking:

> Have you had unsafe sex in the last month?
> Yes/No

Another approach is to word the question so that it is clear that the behaviour is common or not especially uncommon. A question could be phrased: 'Most of us park on double yellow lines occasionally . . .'. For sensitive topics open questions are obviously advantageous. It is also the case that questions on sensitive topics require a longer preamble than those on non-sensitive topics. Again, it is important to use language with which the respondent is familiar, rather than technical language.

A different approach to asking questions about areas where people may not be truthful because of embarrassment is to depersonalize it by putting together a small vignette. Asking about someone else's behaviour and whether or not the respondent approves of it may yield a more truthful answer.

RELIABILITY

In order to be considered reliable a questionnaire should produce broadly the same responses if answered by the same person on another day, or by someone thought to be similar at any time. This is especially important in a longitudinal study, which takes place over a long period of time and where one is looking for change in opinions or behaviour, not change in answering the question. 'Test–retest reliability' can be assessed by repeating the administration of the questionnaire to some of the same subjects after a short interval, e.g. a week or a month.

Internal reliability

This is a means of ascertaining that a person is answering the questionnaire reliably throughout. It involves asking the same question more than once but using different wording, and then checking that the answers mean the same. A directly opposite question can also be used to ensure that the answer given is also opposite. If the answers are inconsistent then the respondent either has not read the questions properly, has not understood them, or has not taken the questionnaire seriously, and in these cases should be regarded as a non-responder.

VALIDITY

A questionnaire is valid if the measurements taken from it reflect the true situation. Validity in newly designed questionnaires is difficult to prove, and the construction of a truly valid questionnaire is probably beyond the scope of this book. One way to improve or to prove the validity of a questionnaire you are designing is to add on well validated instruments, e.g. the General Health Questionnaire, or to use some questions from these in your own questionnaire. Well validated questionnaires are ones which have been through a rigorous process of expert advice and have been used on a number of occasions. These are the types of questionnaire that one can obtain from books of health measures (e.g. Wilkin *et al.* 1992 and Bowling 1991, 1995; see Further reading).

STRUCTURE

The structure of the whole questionnaire and the sequence of the questions within it needs to be thought about carefully. It needs to be made clear to the respondents why the questionnaire is important. This is often done in an accompanying letter rather than on the questionnaire itself. Remember that respondents have to be motivated to spend their own time filling in your questionnaire. The front page or introductory paragraph of the questionnaire should be clear and concise (Box 6.1). A 'funnel design' is usually the most comfortable sequence of questions, moving from the general to the particular. The initial part of the questionnaire should be neutral but interesting, with the more sensitive items appearing later.

Box 6.1 Introduction to the questionnaire
- The aim or purpose of the study is clearly stated, e.g. improvement of a service
- Likely timing is given for completion of the form, e.g. 5–10 minutes
- Reassurances are given concerning confidentiality and anonymity of responses (where appropriate)
- Names of the individuals or organizations involved are given
- A statement is made that failure to complete the questionnaire will not influence your normal standard of care
- How and where the completed questionnaire will be collected is described, e.g. prepaid envelope or box in surgery
- The respondent is always thanked for devoting the time to complete the form
- A contact name and address is clearly marked

Pay attention to the layout of the questionnaire, using clear print and colour when possible – the visual impact of the form is critical, and it has been shown that we are more motivated to complete self-administered questionnaires which have a professional look about them. The questions need to follow a logical sequence: it is very irritating to be asked questions concerning wedding presents if you are actually asked whether you are married or not three questions later. The question about marriage should come first, and should probably be followed by a skip instruction (see below).

Demographic questions – those about age, marital status etc. – have traditionally been put at the beginning of questionnaires, but we would argue for their going at the end as they are relatively personal. They may be potentially less interesting than the questions about your main themes, and may put people off completing the whole questionnaire if they are located at the start, but they are nevertheless extremely important. People may feel that their age and gender, for example, are sensitive topics, or they may simply not see the relevance of these types of questions. If respondents do not give this type of information about themselves you may be unable to analyse meaningfully the main themes of the questionnaire. By and large, questions at the end of a questionnaire are answered because people have already invested time and effort in completing the questionnaire and are motivated to finish.

It is essential to make it absolutely clear that the questionnaire will be confidential.

Do not be tempted to try and make your questionnaire appear shorter by cramming the questions together. It is much more important that the respondent has enough space to answer and that questions are laid out in an understandable form, than that the questionnaire can be completed on one sheet of paper. It is always worth putting a general question at the end of the whole questionnaire, for example, 'is there anything that you would like to add?', as this will sometimes produce information on areas that you had not even thought of.

Skip questions

Most of us are familiar with the sort of question that says 'if yes, go to question 11'. This is a skip question. In order to avoid the respondent missing the directions, the instruction should come after the answer, not after the question. In addition, Sudman and Bradburn (1982) suggest that more errors are made when the skip follows a 'no' response, so skip instructions are best triggered by a 'yes' response.

SENDING

When sending a questionnaire always ensure that the return address is on the questionnaire itself, normally at the end. People lose covering letters, and even envelopes! In the covering letter explain who you are and what you are hoping to discover from the research. Stress confidentiality and the need for as many people as possible to respond. Giving your subject a strong sense of the importance of this work to you ('my degree depends on *your* help') or to medical science ('this could help sick children') can persuade respondents to reply. Doctors may be less altruistic and more self-interested ('the results of this research could help reduce your workload').

Remember to thank your subjects, they are doing you a favour.

If you wish to identify your respondents you will need to have a box in the top right-hand corner of the questionnaire that identifies where it has come from and from which respondent.

BIAS

Bias arises because of the way in which the questions are asked. Respondents will try to give the answer they perceive as being 'socially desirable' or prestigious. Questions need to be framed so that the low-prestige answer is just as acceptable as the high-prestige one.

Respondents will tend to give positive answers. They are also reluctant to use the extreme categories in Likert scales – a central tendency operates. Where ethical or moral standards exist respondents will tend to say they would comply, even if they really would not. In questionnaires where respondents are seeking help they may make the situation worse than it actually is if it seems to be to their advantage.

CODING OF RESPONSES

Coding is the method by which responses to closed questions are converted to numerical data for entry on to computer for analysis. This can be done either by assigning a number to each box that the respondent marks, e.g. *yes = 1, no = 2, don't know = 3*, or by putting boxes in the right-hand margin for someone to go through and complete when the questionnaire is returned. Methods of coding responses should be prepared in advance to make data entry as straightforward as possible. Self-coding, i.e. when the respondent or interviewer codes the responses in the course of completing the questionnaire, is quicker and cheaper than separate coding and reduces the risk of transcription errors. Conventionally a 9 is used to indicate a missing response.

The codes are then entered on to a computer database, which may need to be designed specially, and the advice of a statistician or someone experienced in the design of such coding frames should be sought (Chapter 14). The database can be used to 'clean' the data, that is to check that they have been coded and entered correctly; this is a specialist skill and we would strongly advise you to obtain help to do this.

The coding and analysis of open question responses is covered in Chapters 5 and 7.

RESPONDING

Most biases disappear if a response rate of 70% or more is achieved. However, it is very difficult to achieve such a high rate on a postal questionnaire.

Factors that seem to increase the response rate are:

- Including a stamped addressed envelope
- Including a covering letter from the patient's GP
- Government sponsorship (DoH)
- Incentives, e.g. money!
- A pen.

Factors which do not seem to make any difference:

- Business reply envelope
- Coloured paper or envelope
- Personalizing (Dear Mrs Bloggs)
- An imposing letterhead
- Which day of the week the letter is received
- A first- or second-class stamp (therefore use a second)
- Addressing women as Ms or Mrs
- Signing the letter personally (as opposed to a photocopy)
- The status of the sender
- Asking respondents to tick a box or ring a number.

The factor most likely to increase your response rate is asking about a subject which is of interest to the respondent.

A good questionnaire is one that works. If time and resources permit, repeat your survey at least once. This will allow you to perform validation, to increase sample size and to improve your questions to the point where you are proud of them.

Further reading

Abramson JH (1990) *Survey Methods in Community Medicine.* Churchill Livingstone, Edingburgh.

Armstrong D and Grace J (1994) *Research Methods and Audit in General Practice.* Oxford University Press, Oxford.

Bell J (1993) *Doing Your Research Project.* Open University Press, Buckingham.

Bowling A (1991) *Measuring Health.* Open University Press, Buckingham.

Bowling A (1995) *Measuring Disease.* Open University Press, Buckingham.

Jarman B (1983) Identification of underprivileged areas. *BMJ.* **286**: 1705–9.

Lee RM (1993) *Doing Research on Sensitive Topics.* Sage, London.

Lydeard S (1991) The questionnaire as a research tool. *Family Practice.* **8**(1): 84–91.

May T (1993) *Social Research Issues, Methods and Process.* Open University Press, Buckingham.

Phillimore P, Beattie A and Townsend P (1994) Widening inequality of health in Northern England, 1981–91. *BMJ.* **308**: 1125–8.

Stewart M, Tudiver F, Bass MJ, Dunn EV and Norton PJ (1992) *Tools for Primary Care Research.* Sage Publications, Newbury Park.

Stone DH (1993) How to design a questionnaire. *BMJ.* **307**: 1264–6.

Sudman S and Bradburn NM (1982) *Asking Questions: a Practical Guide to Questionnaire Design.* Jossey-Bass, San Francisco.

Wilkin D, Hallam L and Doggett M-A (1992) *Measures of Need and Outcome for Primary Health Care.* Oxford University Press, Oxford.

7

Coding and analysing data

John Skelton

INTRODUCTION

The great advantage of using open-ended questionnaires and interviews to collect data is that you hand over to people the right to talk about what they want. In just the way that patient-centred consultations are a 'good thing', so respondent-centred data collection is a good thing.

This leads us to the disadvantages, which are obvious but worth pinning down (see Box 7.1 and Tables 7.1 and 7.2). What problems can you see in coding and making sense of these data? Play the sceptic, and before you read on see what you can come up with.

Box 7.1 contains data collected in interviews; Tables 7.1 and 7.2 are sets of open responses to a written questionnaire. The interview invited members of primary health care teams (PHCTs) to talk about episodes of violence and aggression they had been subjected to at work. The questionnaire asked undergraduates to nominate up to three things they enjoyed and three they did not about a role-play course.

A sceptic speaks

Here are some points you might have made in your role as sceptic:

'But it's all just people's ideas, isn't it? I mean "I felt menaced" (Box 7.1 no 1). What does that mean? Some lads were hanging around? Who says that's aggressive?'

This is a key point, in fact, about any person-based data. Even assuming a willingness to be truthful, what you get when you ask people is perceptions of truth, not

---

Box 7.1 Interview data on violence and agression at work

1. I felt so menaced by the people outside the house that I actually delayed the visit. I didn't do the visit, came away, left my car back at the health centre and felt I was better to walk rather than have my car broken into.

2. I find the hardest aggression to deal with is the indirect, say maybe a very well-educated person that you're going in to do something for and it's kind of 'oh well use the back door that's the tradesman's entrance . . .'

3. Five youths went into the antenatal erm clinic erm obviously full of pregnant mums and small babies and they were just playing absolute havoc knocking everything over and that, that's very frightening.

4. The patient is very aggressive and saying four letter words on the telephone to the receptionist and that call was passed on to me . . . they didn't know any other language to exp[lain] erm to say what they g[zz] say it doesn't mean they are aggressive and there's some of them have apologized after . . .

Table 7.1 Negative comments

1	More, shorter, easier role plays to prepare us
2	More role play
3	All good experience
4	More role plays, less lectures
5	Not enough time and opportunity for all to do role play
6	Give more time to give everyone a chance to do role play
7	Too big a group
8	Groups maybe should be smaller so less nervous, more people have a go
	Need more info on cases
9	More role plays after having discussions on them
10	More varied role plays
11	The role plays included a lot of medical knowledge, which we as yet do not know of – this could put us in a bad position at times – looking a fool
12	Some role plays – too much factual info to retain, e.g. testicular cancer
13	Maybe start role playing with easier situations – rather than the first time you get to talk to a stranger in this situation you're telling them their husband died etc.
14	In role play I needed to know more specific details – props, e.g. tissues
15	Some props might be helpful, e.g. box of tissues, cup of tea

---

the thing itself. A great many studies slip illegitimately from 'is reported to be' ('GPs say they are overworked, undervalued and underpaid') to 'is' ('GPs are overworked, undervalued and underpaid'), and this respondent, after all, might easily have said 'I was menaced' rather than 'I felt menaced'. What this piece of data tells us is that

Table 7.2 Positive comments

16	Making me do a role play, even though I didn't want to
17	Small group discussions
18	Role plays
19	The chance to have a go yourself and be evaluated
20	Realistic situations
21	Giving us practice at speaking to 'patients'
22	Role plays – esp. bad news ones
23	Role play
24	Discussion
25	Demonstration
26	Video
27	Role plays
28	Discussion role plays
29	Role play
30	Role play
31	Role play
32	Role plays very useful
33	Role plays with people we've never met is very good
34	Hints on structuring interviews
35	Role play discussions
36	Importance
37	(Use of actors)

the respondent perceived aggression. For all we know, however, just reading this extract, it was a group collecting for the church jumble sale.

'And what's more, people are so nice. Look at Box 7.1, no 2. They're just trying to help the interviewer. Would anyone *really* call that aggressive?'

The willingness of people of all sorts to give pleasing rather than truthful answers in formal and semiformal situations is well known – we all have the experience as schoolchildren of trying to guess what the teacher wants to hear rather than saying what we believe. Although of course the respondent may well be saying something they have long believed.

This particular example also highlights the fact that people use words to mean different things. We might say we're 'angry' about world poverty or missing the bus, but presumably our emotions are not the same. A lot of questionnaire and interview research rests on the presumption that people use words to mean the same thing – that when you and I both say we are 'very dissatisfied' with the latest government initiative we are reflecting a similar degree of irritation, despite the fact that I have a delightfully sunny disposition and everyone knows what an old curmudgeon you are.

'With data like these, you only see what you want to see. Look at Table 7.1, no 1. This might mean lots of things. So how will you interpret it? No, don't tell me, I can guess: you'll find what suits you best.'

Sadly, yes; this might mean the student wants more role play in general, or more of the short easy role plays he or she thinks have happened; or more role plays in general, but specifically so that short and easy ones can be added to the existing range of long and difficult ones. The potential for grammatical ambiguity in questionnaire responses is very considerable.

Researchers do indeed run the risk of finding what they want to find, more generally of being conditioned by their own cultural presumptions and professional training, and more generally still of finding other points of view incomprehensible. An extreme example of this is reported, with pleasing self-mockery, by Skipper and McGahy (1972), who found themselves unable to conduct an effective interview backstage with a stripper. They conclude, 'Our sheltered background and numerous courses in sociological methodology simply had not prepared us for this kind of research environment'.

This is true not only of this kind of study but of science in general. We are all aware of Kuhn's (1962) notion of 'paradigms' (as in: 'there's been a paradigm shift in this practice since I arrived and knocked a few heads together') – of the fact, roughly, that we interpret data according to our predilections (though Kuhn is famously imprecise about his use of the term).

We think as we are trained to think, and find what we are trained to look for. Doctors think like doctors and may interpret data to fit a medical mindset: other people do not. Becker (1971), talking of classroom observation (this is a much explored field in qualitative research), says:

> . . . it takes a tremendous effort of will and imagination to stop seeing only the things that are conventionally "there" to be seen. I have talked to a couple of teams of research people who have sat around in classrooms trying to observe and it is like pulling teeth to get them to see or write anything beyond what "everyone" knows. (p10)

'But the bottom line here is that it's all so wildly subjective. Look at Box 7.1, 3 and 4. How are you going to categorize them? As "the same" or "different"? Is trashing a surgery like swearing down the telephone? What standard of "likeness", precisely, is at issue here . . . particularly as the explicit accusation of aggression in no 4 appears to be subsequently withdrawn?'

Yes, exactly. Some data yield a straightforward choice between a well-accepted set of criteria. Are you male or female? Legally married, single, divorced, widowed? These are categories which all people will understand and which are more or less mutually exclusive, well-defined, and exhaust the possibilities. Virtually nobody (a bigamously married individual in the middle of a sex change?) would have difficulty in confidently ticking the right boxes.

The situation is never like this with open questionnaires and interviews – if it were, they would be unnecessary in the first place. If all truth could be reduced to a set of boxes to tick we would have no need of qualitative research (or the faculty of language, if it comes to that). Typically, in this kind of enquiry the researcher will not be measuring data against a thoroughly validated, mutually exclusive, exhaustive list: rather, he or she will be aware that ambiguity and uncertainty are the name of the game.

So there you are then!

Well, no. The point is that who we are and the experiences we have simply cannot always be clearly categorized, and if we are to tackle them at all we need to be prepared to develop methodologies that can handle the confusing and unsorted bits of our world. Both quantitative and qualitative methodologies have problems with categorization, after all:

> The need to quantify can lead to imposing arbitrary categories on complex phenomena, just as data extraction in qualitative research can be used selectively to tell a story that is rhetorically convincing but scientifically incomplete. (Mays and Pope 1996, p17)

FINDING ORDER IN DATA

Success in uncovering order and pattern in these kinds of data is really a matter of understanding and countering problems.

Two preliminary remarks, however. First, it is seldom possible (or plausible) to set up extensive categories for data of this kind in advance of data collection. Themes arise in the researcher's mind from the study of the data. This can make the researcher feel that the whole study is a bit ad hoc, too disorganized for its own good. But, secondly – an important point – this is typical, and not a cause for concern. The sensation of working with qualitative data is inevitably, and properly, one of exploration and uncertainty, of the slow development of categories which may be obvious or forced on one, of coding decisions tentatively made and abandoned, and then returned to in the end.

Such matters are discussed in the literature and dignified with such names as 'grounded theory' (Glaser and Strauss 1968) in which the research design and the analysis of data proceed side by side, with the latter informing the former, and quite deliberately not being separated from it. One purpose of this chapter is to give the researcher pemission to proceed along these lines, and to recognize that they too are systematic.

This may seem like good news, but it should be borne in mind that there are two drawbacks. First, only very perceptive coding and interpretation is of any value, and secondly, given the discursive rather than numerical basis of the enquiry, articulate exposition is at a premium (many qualitative researchers, particularly the more ethnographically oriented, are in fact extremely good writers).

At any rate, all approaches use a form of content analysis. This phrase, like grounded theory, can refer to a particular set of procedures, such as those outlined in Box 7.2, but I shall use the term less precisely.

The central problem in coding data is this: you can look at the transcripts of 50 interviews on Monday and they all seem to be saying more or less the same thing. Look at them again on Tuesday and they all seem to be saying entirely different things. The question people tend to pose at this stage is, Which viewpoint is right? But a much better question is: For my purposes, what is the most appropriate level of analysis? A hundred categories or one? How *delicate* should my analysis be?

There are two things that can help you. One is to improve the reliability of your data (and your own confidence in it), either by asking someone else to code independently from you, or by checking on the data ('triangulating' it), or some aspect of it, by collecting similar information in a different way.

The other important resource you have is to ask yourself, at all stages, 'What can I predict?' If your first respondent tells you your practice has been tight-fisted since it started fundholding you can shrug your shoulders. If the next five all say the same, you may be forced to acknowledge an emerging pattern, and so on. With interviews it is rare to be getting new information after talking to 30 respondents. When you end up saying 'The next respondent will certainly say X, and will probably say Y', you will know that X and Y are categories you can confidently set up.

Note, however, that it is in the nature of data of this kind to be ambiguous, and for particular pieces of data – what this particular respondent said – to be potentially codifiable under more than one of the categories you set up. There are two possible responses to this: one is to accept that there is a problem, and simply reach a judgement about 'best fit'. In other words, you accept that in the absence of an ideal solution, the most appropriate is good enough. The alternative is a much more descriptive approach, which allows you to enter pieces of data under many different categories. This will not be further discussed here: it implies a more discursive, broadly ethnographic approach than we are concerned with, and would involve us in thinking about a different kind of research methodology.

So, you will look at the data you have collected, you will ideally have someone else look at it and categorize it too, and you will develop categories. You may find that at the outset you will often be thinking in terms of categories that are familiar to you (you are comfortable with the paradigms they reflect). Often, too, as you review and reflect you will find unexpected categories suggesting themselves to you. This kind of move from theory-driven to data-driven categories and back again is entirely typical. And, finally, you may often find that you need to adjust your categories as you go along – all of these shifts and doubts should be accepted as part of the process.

Finally, there are a number of computer programs you can consider which will help you to organize data, of which Nu-dist and Ethnograph are perhaps the best known. Remember, however, that computers are not very bright: they cannot understand your data for you – they merely store it and order it.

> **Box 7.2 Finding order in data**
> - As you study your data, are you seeing beyond the obvious?
> - Is your analysis at a level of delicacy which best suits your research purposes?
> - Have you used some check on your analysis (another researcher? triangulation?)
> - Does your study have predictive value?

CODING DATA – AN ILLUSTRATION

The remainder of this Chapter looks in detail at Tables 7.1 and 7.2, a particular set of data collected at Birmingham University. You might like now, before you read on, to code these data and see to what extent your thought processes resemble those discussed below. (The Table represents a very small sample of the total data – far too small for this kind of enquiry, but ignore this for the moment.)

One hundred and eighty-seven medical students at Birmingham participated in a series of role play sessions designed to improve their consultation skills. They were subsequently given a questionnaire which 134 of them completed and returned. Students were first asked to grade various elements of the course on a Likert scale and then, in a manner which is typical of this sort of educational evaluation, to specify 'three things which you particularly enjoyed' and 'three things which you did not particularly enjoy and would invite us to reconsider'. Note in passing that these two questions are not mirror images of each other. There is an attempt to make students feel more comfortable about criticizing the course by the positive-sounding phrasing of 'invite us to reconsider'. This is obvious enough. Less obvious is the fact that 'particularly enjoyed' means roughly 'enjoyed very much', whereas 'did not particularly enjoy' is a way of describing a lukewarm rather than a negative response. This was a deliberate choice, once more in the hope that it would offer students permission to criticize. It is nevertheless typical of the way in which what seem like easy language choices in the preparation of questions may have the effect of altering the data.

There is, of course, a hidden agenda: this questionnaire, like many, many others, has the surreptitious subtitle 'Didn't we do well?', a fact on which you might like to reflect. Let us concentrate on the negative comments.

Numbers 2 and 3 are, in fact, clearly positive statements, presumably written down at all merely so that the interviewee can demonstrate to the researcher that he or she has seen the question. Presumably we can ignore these comments (of which, in fact, there were a large number in the data). Comment 4 might also be viewed in this category – as a wish for more on another occasion, based purely on present satisfaction. It might equally, however, be put with comments 5 and 6, which clearly seem to suggest, not so much that the course content was excellent as that the time given over to it was ill judged.

Another version of the logistical problem is to criticize not the time available but the number of groups, so that all students could not participate equally fully (comment 7). The respondent for comment 8 also wanted small groups, but the reason is manifestly different: small groups would reduce the extent to which individuals were nervous.

Here, then, is one set of issues about which generalizations need to be made. You might like to set up a general category headed 'Group size and its consequences' and another, 'Time and its consequences'. Or, alternatively, you may want to set up a major heading 'Resourcing issues', with two subheadings: 'Group size' and 'Time'. The issue here is what level of generality you want: did five types of thing happen, or 50? Do we want to see the wood or the trees? Evidently, neither is correct nor incorrect, and there is at least the advantage that the two ways of categorizing this particular piece of data are not mutually inconsistent.

It will be seen that there is a degree of interpretation necessary even with these straightforward responses, an attempt to reconstruct the context that surrounds the words on the page. Written responses are brief.

Another version of the complaint about the inadequate number of role plays is comment 9. This, like a lot of written responses (and like comment 10), verges on grammatical ambiguity. Does the respondent want a greater number of role plays overall, all accompanied by discussion, or a greater proportion of the present number of role plays to be accompanied by discussion? Does the respondent in comment 10 want greater variation in the role plays, or a larger number of those role plays which are already perceived as being varied? Then, as regards discussion, the respondent for comment 12 makes a clear and straightforward point; the respondent for comment 9 may be categorized as either in accord with this point or not.

There is another set of comments (11, 12, 13) which appear to make the same point in a way that would be easy to generalize about. Altogether, seven people seem to make this point. The difficulty here is that when asked directly elsewhere in the questionnaire whether the role-play scenarios were at a clinical level which was 'too hard', 'about right' or 'too easy', no-one said they were too easy; 131 people said they were about right and only three people said that they were too difficult.

Finally, with respect to the negative comments (see Table 7.1), there are issues such as whether to count comment 14 as two comments or one (it seems to make two points), and the appearance of the words 'props' and 'tissues' from two respondents (comments 14 and 15) suggests a degree of contamination of the data, possibly from each other. (On the other hand, I know that one of my colleagues has a standard joke about the use of tissues in role play, which just goes to show how much context a little bit of insider information can give one.)

Now let us consider the positive comments. You will no doubt be able to see evidence here of the points made with regard to the negative comments, so I shall not repeat these. Otherwise, what is most striking is that the data are extremely uninformative. This may be interpreted as the students' inability to be articulate about this particular topic, or it may represent a level of indifference towards the whole questionnaire procedure. It will be seen that the language on display here is very slight – so limited that it is obviously unwise to attempt much interpretation. Apart from this, there are straightforward issues to be resolved, such as whether to include or exclude comment 22, which the respondent has put in parentheses knowing he or she has been asked for a maximum of three comments; and the issue of whether comments 14, 15 or 16, all from the same individual, should be counted as one (presumably they should) or three.

CONCLUSION

The two biggest mistakes that people make about coding and analysing qualitative data are to assume that the whole business is so tenuously validated that it is unscientific, and ought not to be undertaken, and to think it is easy. The difficulty lies in being sensitive to the ambiguities of what is collected, and to the complex contexts from which it arises, but it is this sensitivity which makes the best of such studies scientific and therefore enlightening.

Further reading

Abramson JH (1990) *Survey Methods in Community Medicine*. Churchill Livingstone, London.

Becker HS (1971) Comment in Wax M, Diamond S and Gearing F (eds), *Anthropological Perspectives on Education*. Basic Books, New York.

Glaser BG and Strauss AL (1968) *The Discovery of Grounded Theory: Strategies for qualitative research*. Weiderfeld and Nicholson, London.

Hammersley M and Atkinson P (1993) *Ethnography: Principles in Practice*. Routledge, London.

Kuhn TS (1962) *The Structure of Scientific Revolutions*. University of Chicago Press, Chicago.

Mays M and Pope C (eds) (1996) *Qualitative Research in Health Care*. BMJ, London.

Skipper JK and McGaghy CH (1972) Respondents' intrusion upon the situation: the problem of interviewing subjects with special qualities. *Sociological Quarterly*. **13**: 237–43.

8

Epidemiology and interpreting research studies

Dawood Dassu and Sue Wilson

This chapter aims to introduce, in a non-technical manner, some of the important issues involved in the design and interpretation of studies in which numerical data are collected. Epidemiology is a wide-ranging field and the mere mention of statistics stops many potential researchers from pursuing their own topics of interest. It is hoped that this text will dispel some of the mystique. We present some of the more common types of analysis and discuss general issues relating to the interpretation of research studies. Unfortunately, it is beyond the scope of this short chapter to discuss even this limited range of issues in detail; however, there are many excellent texts that do so. Some of these are listed at the end of the chapter and we strongly recommend the reader to consult them before embarking on their own research project.

WHAT IS EPIDEMIOLOGY?

Clinical medicine is concerned with the individual; in epidemiology the focus is on the population. A *population* comprises *all* individuals with one or more common characteristics, and can range from the general to the specific (e.g. all people resident in the UK, or all asthmatics under five years of age on the list of one specific GP). Epidemiology has been defined as 'the study of the *distribution* and *determinants* of disease *frequency*' (Hennekens and Buring 1987).

The questions tackled by epidemiologists all attempt to quantify, in some way, the distribution, determinants or frequency of morbidity, mortality or some other health-related index, and include:

- *Describing the distribution.* What is the extent of the problem? Who is affected? When and where does it manifest itself in a population? Is this disease more common now than ten years ago? How does the frequency of disease in my practice compare with that in the general population?
- *Identifying the determinants.* Can we identify factors that cause a disease, or are they simply associated with it?
- *Evaluating.* Is policy A more effective than policy B? Is the new policy the most cost-effective? How is patient satisfaction affected by the new policy? Evaluating the effectiveness of screening
- *Surveillance.* Identification of new or changing health care needs. Monitoring existing health care systems or activities. Is this system serving the needs of this community? Can we do it more cost-effectively?
- *Investigating* the natural history of a disease. Can we identify improved methods of prevention, diagnosis or treatment?

Although these questions all have different aims, each is a measurement exercise of some form. Four main types of study are employed, depending on what measurements need to be made: these study designs are discussed in the next section.

STUDY DESIGN

For any researcher the most difficult decision is in choosing the appropriate study design. The more common study designs and some of their main strengths and weaknesses are described below.

Descriptive studies

Cross-sectional

Cross-sectional studies (surveys) usually gather information at one point in time or over a relatively short period. Such studies are primarily used for descriptive purposes; however, a descriptive study may often lead to the generation of hypotheses which will subsequently be tested by more formal studies (e.g. randomized controlled trials, cohort or case control studies). Cross-sectional studies are not always descriptive (e.g. prevalence of coughs in children) and analytical studies can, in some circumstances, be undertaken (e.g. association between coughs in children and exposure to indoor pollutants).

Important issues:

- Surveys that require the respondent to recall events which may have occurred a considerable time ago, are prone to recall bias
- A particular problem of postal questionnaires is non-response. Efforts should be made to maximize the response rate (e.g. reposting and telephone reminders). Non-respondents tend to be atypical, so bias is possible in studies even with high response rates. The characteristics of non-respondents should be recorded and compared to those of respondents before conclusions are made. The various types of bias that can affect research projects are discussed in more detail later in this chapter.

Example 1

A postal questionnaire-based survey of 492 postmenopausal women investigated their knowledge of and attitudes to hormone replacement therapy. One of the study's results is shown below.

	Number	% of responders	% of total sample
Considered HRT	111	25.9	22.6
Never considered	317	74.1	64.4
Did not respond	64		13.0
Total	492		100

Adapted from Sinclair HK, Bond CM, Taylor RJ (1993) Hormone replacement therapy: a study of women's knowledge and attitudes. *Br J Gen Prac.* **43**(374): 365–70.

If this study had been undertaken to inform future policy and the authors had, prior to the commencement of the study, decided that if more than 25% of people had considered HRT it would *not* be worth undertaking a planned health education campaign, then the first column of results might have made them decide that public awareness of HRT was sufficiently high (26%) and no further action was required. However, it is possible that the 64 women who did not respond did not want to admit that they had no knowledge of HRT, and a more realistic estimate of those women who have considered this treatment might be 23%, thus making the planned campaign viable.

If a comparison between two groups (e.g. those with and without disease) is to be made, then it is important that all groups are well represented in the sample, even if some groups are over-represented in relation to their occurrence in the population.

Example 2

A study may wish to look at factors associated with the fictitious blackberry disease. If blackberry disease only occurs once in every 100 people (i.e. affects 1% of the population) then a random sample of 100 people is likely to contain only one case of blackberry disease. Since this single case is unlikely to be representative of all patients with blackberry disease, a comparison of the characteristics (age, sex, hobbies, occupation, diet etc.) of the person with the disease against the 99 without it is unlikely to provide any useful data.

Although the event of interest affects only 1% of the population, a more useful study would compare the characteristics of 50 people with the disease and 50 people without it (case control study).

In cross-sectional studies information on the factors that may be associated with the event of interest, and information on the event itself, are recorded at the same time. However, the event may have occurred before the exposure, and therefore the event and exposure cannot be causally linked. The aetiological significance of associations found in cross-sectional studies depends on how well current exposure correlates with the causal exposure. Such correlation is especially difficult in dietary studies. More reliance can be placed on associations between outcomes and unchanging factors such as ethnic or cultural background and sex.

Example 3
A cross-sectional study may show lower levels of serum β-carotene in cancer patients than in persons not affected with cancer. However, with cross-sectional data it is not possible to say whether the deficiency preceded the onset of cancer or is a result of it.

Measures of frequency: rates

The most basic measures are counts of the number of new (incident) or existing (prevalent) events of interest. However, if study measurements are to be compared with those from another series or population, it is necessary to know the size of the population in which the events occurred and the length of the reporting period.

Precise definitions of the numerator (events of interest) and denominator (population studied) are required. This is particularly important when events or the sample population are difficult to recognize or define.

Prevalence rates summarize the proportion of the population with the disease of interest during a given period of time:

$$\text{Prevalence rate} = \frac{\text{number of existing cases}}{\text{size of population in defined time period}}$$

The prevalence rate is an estimate of the probability that an individual is diseased at a defined period of time. This is a useful measure, especially for chronic conditions. However, estimates of prevalence are dependent on the assumptions made concerning the point in time when a person moves from a 'disease present' to a 'disease absent' state.

Incidence rates describe the proportion of the population that develop the disease of interest during a defined period of time:

$$\text{Incidence rate} = \frac{\text{number of new cases}}{\text{size of population in defined time period}}$$

Example 4: Calculation of incidence rates

	Numerator	Components of the denominator	
Practice	Consultations/cases	Reporting period	List size
A	19	24 months	6000
B	11	12 months	4500

Practice A has more consultations than practice B, but it also has a larger list and a longer reporting period.

Assuming each consultation is a case, for Practice B, dividing the number of cases by the list size will give us the number of cases per individual for one year of observation (11/4500 = 0.00244 per person per year).

For Practice A, the population of 6000 persons has been observed for two years, equivalent to 12 000 people being observed for one year, and the calculation of the rate per year accounts for this (19/(6000 × 2) = 0.0016).

A rate per person is often difficult to comprehend and the rates per individual are usually multiplied by 1000 or 100 000, to calculate rates per 1000 or per 100 000 population.

The annual rates per 1000 for Practice A are 1.58 per 1000 persons per year, and for Practice B 2.44 per 1000 persons per year. These rates could also be expressed in terms of risk, e.g. we would expect 1.58 in every 1000 persons in Practice A to consult each year.

Relative risk: comparing the rate of disease in two populations

Example 4 illustrates how the incidence rate provides a measure of the risk of disease. The ratio of two incidence rates provides the relative risk (RR) of an event occurring in one population compared to another:

$$\text{Relative risk} = \frac{\text{Incidence rate A}}{\text{Incidence rate B}}$$

Relative risks are often used to compare a population exposed to a suspected risk factor with a control population. An RR close to 1.0 suggests no association between exposure and disease; conversely, RRs further from 1.0 (above or below) suggest an association.

Example 5: Calculation of relative risk

Using the data provided for Example 4, the risk of consultation in Practice A relative to the risk in practice B is:

$$\text{Relative risk} = 1.58/2.44$$
$$= 0.65$$

i.e. the risk of consultation for patients on the list of Practice A is 35% less than in Practice B.

Other measures

In some studies the measurements derived may not be of distinct events such as morbidity, but clinical measurements (e.g. systolic blood pressure or serum cholesterol levels), measurements of attitude (1–4 for 'Important' to 'Not important'), or quality of life measures. For such data averages can be calculated and compared or correlation coefficients used.

Standardization

The incidence of many diseases varies with age and sex. Differences in the age/sex structure of different populations, or of the same population over time, may prohibit the use of crude (all ages combined) rates for comparative purposes.

For example, if we wished to compare the incidence of senile dementia in two practices and one practice population is younger than the other, then even if the age-specific incidence rates are the same, more cases will arise in the older population than in the younger. To compare the pattern of disease in the two practices, or in the same practice at different times, it is important to allow for differing population age structures. This is accomplished by age standardization. There are two methods of age standardization in general use, direct and indirect. The one to be used will depend on the comparison required, e.g. each practice with the region, or comparisons between practices. Hennekens and Buring (1987) explain these ideas in more detail, with examples.

Randomized controlled trials

The most basic trial design involves two groups or 'treatment arms'. Consenting individuals are randomly allocated to one of the two arms, which are defined according to the treatment they will receive. In drug trials, for instance, one arm would receive a new treatment and the other a placebo or standard treatment. At the end of the trial the groups are compared in relation to predefined outcome measures. Such trials are referred to as randomized controlled trials (RCTs).

Important issues:

- The goal of randomization is to select groups that are similar in relation to known and unknown demographic, biological or environmental factors that may have a bearing on the outcome. If the groups are identical in all respects, apart from the treatment, then observed differences in outcome can be attributed to the treatment alone
- Without appropriate control groups, it may be found that people may have recovered without intervention. For instance, if a group of asthma patients was treated in the traditional manner for one year and then self-managed for the following year, a comparison of antibiotic use during the two years could not separate the effect of different management strategies from other

factors, such as weather conditions. In a controlled trial the traditional treatment group acts as a control: factors other than treatment should affect both groups equally

- During trials individuals may discontinue taking the treatment they were randomized to (non-compliance), withdraw from the study, or have incomplete data for analysis (withdrawals and incomplete evaluations). Such protocol deviations should be monitored and minimized, as they must be allowed for in the analysis and, if too common, may prevent meaningful comparison
- Wherever possible the patient, physician and researchers should be 'blind' to the treatment allocation. This reduces the possibility of pretrial prejudices biasing the evaluation.

Example 6

A comparison of guided self-management and traditional treatment of asthma is a recent example of an RCT in a primary care setting. The results of comparing the two groups with respect to two outcome measures are shown below.

Outcome measure	Self-management (56 patients)	Traditional treatment (59 patients)	Significance (*P* value)
1 or more unscheduled visits to ambulatory care (outpatients clinics or primary care)	17 (30%)	28 (48%)	0.06
1 or more courses of oral antibiotics	14 (25%)	29 (49%)	0.008

Adapted from Herrola J *et al.* (1996) Randomized comparison of guided self management and traditional treatment of asthma over one year. *BMJ.* **312**: 748–52.

The self-management group experienced fewer episodes of both outcome measures, suggesting that self-management is better than the traditional treatment at reducing the need for ambulatory care and antibiotics.

Cohort studies

In a *prospective* cohort study data are gathered on exposure (exposed/non-exposed/varying levels of exposure) to a suspected risk factor of a group (cohort) of individuals. The cohort is then followed up over time and compared in relation to the occurrence of predefined outcome measure(s). In *retrospective* cohort studies information on exposure and outcome is collected after both have occurred.

Important issues:

- A cohort study can be viewed as a non-randomized clinical trial where exposure is the intervention. In both RCTs and cohort studies the aim is to make all groups as similar as possible, except in respect of the exposure or treatment. Stratified randomization in clinical trials enables a reasonable balance between the groups with respect to important prognostic characteristics. This is not possible in cohort studies, so it is vital that information on known confounders is recorded (see below)

- The number of subjects can be reduced by comparing the exposed group with the general population. Such comparisons may be prone to bias if the exposure is fairly common or the exposed cohort is not comparable with the population
- If the events of interest are rare, then sufficient events will only be observed if prospective cohort studies follow up large groups of individuals. If the event of interest does not occur for a considerable time after exposure, the subjects must be followed up for a long period. Such studies are therefore often time-consuming and expensive
- In historical or retrospective cohort studies information relating to exposure and confounders is determined from historical records. As there no is waiting for outcomes to manifest, there are considerable savings in time and expense; however, there may be inaccurate or incomplete recording of exposure and confounding
- Cohort studies and observational studies are prone to difficulties in selecting appropriate controls. Individuals not currently exposed may have been exposed in the past
- Analysis should be in terms of new events observed. Those events occurring at the early stages of the observation period are excluded, as they may represent disease that was present prior to the commencement of the study but not yet diagnosed.

Example 7
We may hypothesize that chewing gum prevents dyspepsia.

A prospective cohort design would use a representative group of people (such as a random sample of all patients on a GP's list) and ask them to keep a weekly record of the amount and type of gum they chewed. After a defined period of time and when enough cases of dyspepsia have been identified, the exposure levels (to gum) of the dyspeptics can be compared to those of the non-dyspeptics.

Case control studies

In case control studies cases (individuals with the disease) and controls (individuals without the disease) are identified. Information is collected on the characteristics (age, sex, place of residence etc.) and exposure of both groups to suspected risk factors. After adjusting for any variability, which may be related to the outcome of interest, in the characteristics of the groups, the cases and controls are then compared in relation to their experience of exposure. If exposure is higher among the cases, then exposure may be a risk factor; if lower, it may be protective.

Example 8

Doll and Hill's (1950) study into the link between lung cancer and smoking is an early example of a case control study. This study used lung cancer patients as the cases and patients with diseases other than lung cancer as controls. The explanatory variable was whether or not the individual smoked. Data from a preliminary report are presented below.

	Number (%) smokers	Number (%) non-smokers	P value
Males			
Cases of lung cancer	647 (99.7%)	2 (0.3%)	0.00000064
Controls	622 (95.8%)	27 (4.2%)	

Adapted from Doll R and Hill AB (1950) Smoking and carcinoma of the lung. Preliminary report. *BMJ*. **ii**: 739–48.

Although most men included in this study were classified as smokers, the proportion of cases who smoked (99.7%) was higher than the corresponding proportion of controls (95.8%). The extremely small P value indicates that it is unlikely that the observed difference was due to chance alone (P values are discussed in more detail later in this chapter).

Important issues:

- It is vital that cases and controls are selected independently of their exposure status. Otherwise it is possible that cases are selected *because* they are exposed, and controls are selected *because* they are not exposed
- Cases should be defined precisely. Are the cases incident or prevalent? Prevalent cases may have changed their exposure as a consequence of being a case
- Case control studies are useful for studying rare diseases, as all known cases can be included in the study
- The source of the cases should be known. If the cases are not representative of all cases in the population, then the study results cannot be generalized to the total population
- The choice of appropriate controls (matching) is important. Wherever possible, controls should be selected from the same source as the cases
- Observer bias is possible where exposure information is recorded differently for cases and controls, e.g. if the observer is aware of the hypothesis and the case/control status of the individual
- Responder bias occurs in situations where cases and controls recall events differently. Cases, for instance, tend to be more eager to volunteer information
- The advantages of case control studies include that they are relatively cheap and quick to undertake, information can be collected to assess the effect of a wide range of potential risk factors, and they are useful for studying rare events
- The disadvantages include the possibility of selection or observer bias, and difficulties in assessing the sequence of events.

INTERPRETATION OF RESULTS – THE ROLE OF BIAS, CONFOUNDING AND CHANCE

A major part of the interpretation of results from all research studies involves seeking alternative explanations for the findings. For instance, consider a general practitioner who observes eight new cases of childhood leukaemia in a three-year period, whereas in the previous six years he had seen only one. The GP may believe that pollution from a waste incinerator built four years ago is to blame, and he has observed an apparent association between exposure to pollution and leukaemia. Before he can claim to have found 'proof' of a causal link he must first consider whether the statistical association is valid, whether other studies support the hypothesis, and whether the association is biologically plausible.

Inference from even the most carefully designed and executed studies can be affected by chance, bias or confounding. Evidence from all studies should be critically evaluated, with respect to these three alternative explanations, before reaching conclusions or making policy changes.

Bias

Bias or systematic error is always a possible explanation for perceived associations. There are many types of bias and they can enter a study at different times and from different sources. Some types of bias are more important in certain design strategies than others – these are mentioned above in the outlines of design strategies. Here we discuss the two broad types of selection bias and information bias.

Selection bias results in samples that are not representative of the target population, and can arise in numerous ways, the most obvious being that a representative sample was not selected at the outset or inconsistent criteria were applied when selecting cases or controls (sampling bias). It may also arise when there are differences between participants and non-participants (non-response bias). During clinical trials and longitudinal studies individuals who discontinue participation or who are lost to follow-up may differ from the remaining group (dropout bias). The target population may be different from the population at large (e.g. hospital patients or manual workers), and comparisons involving such groups must be cautiously interpreted (membership bias).

Information or observation bias arises when non-comparable information is obtained from different groups of the study sample. Its source can be interviewers or data collectors eliciting or recording information differently for different groups (interviewer bias), or from cases systematically recalling information differently from controls. For example, if the link between cancer and exposure to industrial pollutants is being studied in a case control study and in both cases the interviewer is aware of the hypothesis, and of the diagnosis, both may seek evidence of exposure more enthusiastically than when interviews are conducted with the control group.

Bias should be considered at all stages of the study and its effects minimized by means of careful study design or, where possible, adjustment during analysis. Non-compliance and dropout rates should be frequently monitored and information on the characteristics of these groups should be collected. If withdrawals form a substantial proportion of the sample and significant differences between them and the participating groups are found, the impact of the effect of their exclusion on the results should be explored.

Confounding

The concept of confounding is critical to all research. A confounding variable is one that is associated with the exposure under investigation and independently affects the risk of developing disease, although this principle is universal and not restricted to disease and exposure. The importance of confounding can be illustrated by the following example.

Example 9

It is known that:

- Smoking and lung cancer are associated.
- Alcohol consumption and smoking are associated.

It is hypothesized that:

- Excessive alcohol consumption leads to an increased risk of lung cancer.

In a study aiming to investigate the association between alcohol consumption and lung cancer it is vital to take account of the link between alcohol consumption and smoking, as an apparent association between lung cancer and alcohol could simply be due to the confounding effect of smoking. In this case smoking is a confounding variable.

When evaluating apparent associations one should always question whether the observed effect may be due to confounding. Statistical techniques should be used to adjust for the effect of confounders. In clinical trials the experimenter can, to some extent, control allocation so that the experimental groups are balanced with respect to important confounders, and in relatively large studies random allocation should give balanced groups. However, in observational studies this is not possible, so the recording of and adjustment for confounding variables is essential.

A major function of statistics is to adjust for the effect of confounding factors. Adjustment in studies with only a few categorical variables, such as sex and social class, can be relatively straightforward (stratified analysis). Analysis of more complex studies may require more sophisticated statistical methods. The principle underlying all methods aiming to adjust for the effect of confounding is to compare like with like. For instance, if age is known to be a risk factor, and exposure to a suspected risk factor differs by age, the analysis would include separate measures of the risk of disease by age group.

Sample size: the role of chance

Research questions usually relate to large groups of individuals, e.g. non-insulin dependent diabetics, or asthmatic children under five years of age. However, such populations are usually too large or ill-defined for information to be collected on *every* member. Therefore, a relatively small sample from the population is selected for study, the assumption being that results from the sample can be extended to the population. It is, however, inevitable that the composition and characteristics of samples will differ from each other owing to chance or sampling variation: samples chosen on different occasions or from different locations will not be identical to each other. Larger samples can generally be relied upon more than smaller ones; the larger the sample, the more likely we are to represent the total population. It must be remembered, however, that no inference based on a sample is infallible. P values, calculated in tests of statistical significance, help us quantify the extent to which our extension from the sample to the population may be due to chance. The interpretation of P values and related confidence intervals is discussed in more detail below.

Establishing the size of the sample required to produce meaningful results is an important part of the study design. Results from studies that are too small will involve too much uncertainty; studies that are unnecessarily large will waste resources. In general, studies should be large enough to have a good chance of detecting clinically significant differences with an acceptable degree of certainty. Prior to estimating the sample size the researcher must have formulated an appropriate study design, have some idea of the smallest clinically significant effect and, in the case of continuous outcome measures, the variability (standard deviation) of the measure.

A sample size calculation yields an estimate of the minimum number of subjects required to give the study a reasonably high probability ('power') of detecting a clinically meaningful effect (if it truly exists), at a statistically significant level. Pocock (1983) provides examples and formulae for sample size calculations, and Lwanga (1991) provides preprepared tables of sample sizes for different study designs.

The 'scientific' requirement for large sample sizes will often have to be balanced against the practical limitations of resources and the availability of cases. It is important to remember that well designed yet small trials can be useful in generating information that may not provide conclusive results but can be used to justify the need for, and assist with the design of, larger trials that will provide more definitive answers.

TESTS OF STATISTICAL SIGNIFICANCE: P VALUES AND CONFIDENCE INTERVALS

Tests of statistical significance are used to quantify the role of chance. The logic of a test is as follows:

1. Assume there is no effect – the population means or proportions that we wish to compare are the same. This assumption is known as the null hypothesis.

2. Find the probability of observing the effect (mean, proportion etc.) estimated by this study, or one more extreme, given the assumption in (1).

3. If that probability (P value) is 'small' it is unlikely that the observed effect is due to chance; in other words, the alternative hypothesis is more tenable than the null hypothesis. The alternative hypothesis is that there is an effect.

This logic is analogous to the situation in a court of law, where the defendant is innocent until proven guilty (null hypothesis). A P value reflects the degree of evidence against the null hypothesis.

Small or 'significant' P values (by convention, less than 5%) indicate that chance is an unlikely explanation for the observed effect, they are not 'proof' of an effect. An important part of the process of interpreting significant P values is to ask 'Does the effect make sense?' If there is no reasonable scientific explanation for a significant result, then the possibility that it may be spurious should be considered.

Example 6 revisited

If the comparison of guided self-management and traditional treatment of asthmatics had also undertaken age-specific analyses, we would not be surprised to see that the requirement for oral antibiotics increased with age.

However, if there was a significantly reduced requirement for oral antibiotics only in those aged 40–54, and there was no physiological explanation or a priori reason for this, then it is possible that the result is merely an artefact of the data.

The size of the P value depends on the sample size and the size of the effect.

Example 6 revisited

In the trial of self-management of asthma the comparison of visits to ambulatory care yielded $P = 0.06$ (6%). This does not mean there is no difference between self-management and traditional treatment with respect to ambulatory care visits. If the same proportions were found in a trial with more patients, or the effect was larger, this difference would translate to a P value less than 6% and be deemed 'significant'. A P value of 6% reflects a marginally greater degree of uncertainty over the authenticity of the effect than a P value of 5%.

The validity of a P value also depends on whether the assumptions underlying the appropriate statistical test are valid. Moreover, P values should be interpreted in conjunction with clinical significance. An effect can be statistically significant but clinically insignificant (i.e. too small to warrant a change in policy). Once an effect has been estimated, both its clinical and statistical significance should be assessed by calculating confidence intervals.

Example 10

Wald *et al.* estimated that two-view mammography detects 24% more cases of breast cancer than one-view mammography. The 95% confidence interval around the estimate is from 16% to 31%. So, although 24% is the best estimate of the effect of two-view mammography, effects from 16% to 31% are also plausible. The true effect is unlikely to be worse than 16%, and equally unlikely to be better than 31%.

If an increased detection rate of breast cancers of 16% is judged to be clinically significant, then the results of this study are sufficient to suggest a change in breast screening policy.

The wider the confidence interval the greater the uncertainty about the true value of the effect.

Example 10 revisited

If the *P* value still suggests evidence of an effect ($P < 0.05$) but the 95% confidence interval covers a wider range, including small and unimportant effects, then there is even less certainty as to the true effect being around 24%. Such a situation could have arisen if, say, only a quarter of the study sample had been used, all other things being equal, the confidence interval would then have ranged from around 8% to 38%.

If this study had been conducted on the smaller sample and the results showed that two-view mammography detected 24% more cases of breast cancer, but the lower range of the 95% confidence interval was only 8%, then there might not be sufficient justification to advocate a change in policy.

A wide variety of statistical tests exist to suit the different types of data that are collected – continuous, categorical, ranked etc. For the more numerate researcher introductory texts on medical statistics may be useful for selecting the appropriate test; for others, the preferred option may be to seek statistical advice.

ANALYSIS

One area we have not discussed is data analysis. We are of the opinion that if a study is well designed and conducted then the analysis is usually a relatively simple matter. A well designed study can yield valid conclusions on the basis of simple analyses (e.g. cross-tabulations, plots, means, standard deviations and simple tests of statistical significance). Some investigators will wish to seek statistical advice with respect to the analysis of their data, but others will feel able to perform the analysis themselves. However, it must be stressed that a common mistake is to collect the data and then consult a statistician about the analysis. Statisticians can advise on the design of studies as well as their analysis, and their advice should be sought at the early stages of a project. Early consultation leads to more fruitful collaboration, as the statistician will have agreed the aims and design of the study and be more appreciative of the context of the data. On this cautionary note, no amount of statistical analysis – no matter how sophisticated – can rescue a poorly designed and executed study.

This chapter has attempted to discuss some of the issues concerning study design and interpretation of results in a non-statistical manner. Our intention has been to illustrate the variety of approaches available to describe or investigate health and disease in the primary care setting. We have not attempted to provide a textbook that will enable a member of the primary care team to begin a research study, but rather to demystify some of the terminology and reference some of the existing textbooks that discuss the issues in more depth and in a user-friendly fashion.

Further reading

Abramson JH (1990) *Survey Methods in Community Medicine: Epidemiological Studies, Programme Evaluation, Clinical Trials*, 4th edn. Churchill Livingstone, London.

Armitage P and Berry G (1994) *Statistical Methods in Medical Research*, 3rd edn. Blackwell Scientific Publications, Oxford.

Bland M (1987) *An Introduction to Medical Statistics*. Oxford University Press, Oxford.

BMA (1993) *Epidemiology for the Uninitiated*, 3rd edn. British Medical Association, London.

Gore SM and Altman DG (1982) *Statistics in Practice*. British Medical Association, London.

Hennekens CH and Buring JE (1987) *Epidemiology in Medicine*. Little, Brown and Company, Boston/Toronto.

Lwanga SK (1991) *Sample Size Determination in Health Studies: a Practical Manual*. World Health Organization, Geneva.

Pocock SJ (1983) *Clinical Trials: a Practical Approach*. John Wiley & Sons, Chichester.

Wald NJ, Murphy P, Major P *et al.* (1995) UKCCCR Multicentre randomized controlled trial of one and two-view mammography in breast cancer screening. *BMJ.* **311**: 1189–92.

9

Research ethics committees

Martin Kendall and Yvonne Carter

INTRODUCTION

The work of the local research ethics committee (LREC) is based on the concern that whereas 'the community needs knowledge, the patient or volunteer needs protection'. It is clear that to advance our understanding of health and disease with the aim of improving health care, we need to make observations, collect data and do research. However, we must at the same time respect the rights of the patients or volunteers and ensure that the risks of harm, distress or inconvenience are acceptable. The research ethics committee is therefore set up to make value judgements about the nature of the research and the impact on the persons being studied. Unfortunately, the researcher driven by the desire or the need to do research may underestimate (consciously or unconsciously) the problems faced by the patient or volunteer, whereas a lay patient support group may fail to understand the potential benefits of the research and exaggerate the unwanted effects on the individual in the study. An independent group consisting of both medical scientists who understand the nature of the project and lay and other members who try to see things from the patient's point of view, is therefore set up to try to find the right balance.

The researcher needs to know of the existence of the LREC, must understand what they are appointed to do, and must consult them about any research which has an impact on people. The decision about which projects need LREC approval will be considered later, but in simple terms when there is a choice for the patient to do A or B, or even to do or not to do A (for example fill in a form or attend a clinic), or for the investigator to do X or Y to the patient, this is research. Audit, which may be considered a form of research, usually involves observing, documenting or evaluating clinical practice, and usually has no immediate impact on the patient, although it may highlight practices which need to be changed, which in turn may have an impact on the patient at a later stage.

There are at least four good reasons why LREC approval should be sought. First, the committee is usually very experienced and may well ask questions and make suggestions which may make the project scientifically more rigorous, but, more importantly, make things easier, more understandable and safer for the patient. This is not only humane and right, but is also more likely to ensure that the study runs smoothly. Secondly, if anything goes wrong and LREC approval has not been obtained, the legal, financial and other consequences will be very much more serious. Thirdly, most journals will not publish papers based on studies that have not been approved by an LREC. Finally, although there is no legal requirement to obtain approval, the Department of Health has stated that LRECs 'should consider the ethical implications of all research proposals which involve human subjects . . .'. This view is universally supported by all the major national bodies involved in regulating medical conduct.

A HISTORICAL PERSPECTIVE

A brief study of history, literature and even the daily news programmes is sufficient to draw attention to 'man's inhumanity to man'. In many instances the damage done is deliberate, and this was true of some of the scientific experiments performed in the concentration camps during the Second World War. However, in medical research patients and volunteers may suffer in a variety of ways, because the researcher underestimates the effects of what is proposed, fails to see the project from the patient's point of view, and does not treat the patient with the concern and consideration due to a fellow human being. Over the last 30 years attitudes have changed and respect for the patient and the volunteer has improved considerably, and this is due in large part to the impact of LRECs. However, the ways in which LRECs work and the framework in which they work still need a great deal of attention.

The improvements achieved in the way in which human subjects are treated in medical research projects are the consequence of a series of publications and events, which include:

● The Declaration of Helsinki, first adopted by the World Medical Assembly in Finland in June 1964 and amended at subsequent meetings of the assembly in Venice (1983) and Hong Kong (1989). The document contains a series of sensible and humane proposals and is frequently incorporated into protocols for major studies. Thus the researchers specify that they will be guided by the principles of the Declaration of Helsinki. One particular sentence states that 'concern for the interests of the subject must always prevail over the interests of science and society'.

- *Human Guinea Pigs: Experimentation in Man* by M. H. Pappworth (1967). This book drew attention to the work which had been published in previous years in which patients had been studied in a way the author considered unethical. At the time medical researchers felt very vulnerable and tried to play down the book's findings. However, the book indicated that the principles of the Declaration of Helsinki were not being put into practice. It made a big impact, and medical research methods had to change.
- Department of Health – *Local Research Ethics Committees* (1991). By this time most district health authorities had set up ethics committees. This document formalized the guidelines indicating who should be on ethics committees, how they should work, and also offered guidance in relation to certain specific problems, such as research on the fetus, children, women and prisoners.
- The *British Medical Journal*, 9 September 1995. This issue contained an editorial on local research ethics committees, by Professor Alberti, which clearly summarized the historical aspects and the problems facing these committees. The same issue contained three other papers on the problems produced by the way ethics committees work, and one on the potential role of an ethics committee to offer guidance in relation to clinical problems.

LOCAL RESEARCH ETHICS COMMITTEES

These are set up by and are the responsibility of the district health authority. They are a little variable in their constitution and in the way they work, but they base their activities on the guidance given by the Royal College of Physicians in a document published in 1990, the Department of Health guidelines (1991) and the results of a study published for the King's Fund Institute by Julia Neuburger in 1992.

The committee should have 8–12 members and should include:

- Hospital medical staff
- Nursing staff
- A general practitioner
- Two or more lay people.

It is suggested that either the chairperson or the vice chairperson should be a lay member. In practice, the chairperson is usually medical as it is helpful for someone who understands the research to lead the meetings and to provide advice on what needs to be submitted to the committee and how it should be presented.

The committee may also include:

- A pharmacist
- A priest
- A lawyer
- A clinical pharmacologist.

Submissions are usually made on forms designed by the committee to enable them to find out what they want easily. Unfortunately, there is no standardization, so that applications to multiple LRECs require many different forms to be filled in.

MAKING AN APPLICATION

The LREC is not a panel of experts and therefore the application should be written in a language which will be understood by an intelligent lay person.

The committee will want to know a number of different things:

About the project:

- What you want to do
- Why you want to do it
- How you will do it
- Where you will do it
- Who will be involved and do they have the expertise?
- Will nurses or other colleagues be involved, and if so do they know all about the study?

About any drug to be used:

- Is it a marketed preparation, is it currently being investigated, or is it a new entity?
- What information is available on its safety, and particularly how many volunteers and patients have been given the drug and did it have any serious adverse effects?
- Is it likely to upset the patient?
- Will a comparator drug or a placebo be used?
- Where will the drug be stored, who will dispense it, and do the pharmacists know about the trial?

About other procedures, investigations:

- Are these safe?
- Are they necessary?
- Is radiation involved? If so, how much and has appropriate advice on its safe use been obtained?

About the patients and volunteers:

- How will these be selected?
- Are they really volunteers or is there any kind of pressure? Is it absolutely certain that no untoward consequences (delays, suboptimal treatment, for example) will result if the patient does not wish to take part?

- Will any risk to the patient be minimized by appropriate selection and by ensuring that those doing the study are competent and the place in which it is done is suitable (i.e. enough space to lay the patient down, to allow access by medical staff if needed) and that there is equipment and drugs to resuscitate the patient if necessary?
- Has the patient/volunteer given informed consent (see below)?

About legal and financial aspects:

- Are there adequate arrangements to compensate the patient or respond to legal claims should the need arise?
- How is the study funded, and are patients being harmed or inconvenienced to provide the investigators with cash or other rewards?

INFORMED CONSENT

An LREC will want to know how you intend to obtain informed consent. This is critically important, as if a mentally normal, conscious adult understands fully what is involved in a study, and freely agrees to take part, then most of the ethics committee's concerns will have been addressed. The problems are to determine what is required to give informed consent, and to decide what is meant by consent freely given.

The patient can, and probably should, be informed both verbally and in writing. However, it is the written information that will be submitted to the LREC. In some countries where the risk of litigation is high, and for some international drug companies, the only way to fully inform the patient is with a large, detailed document. This is often unintelligible and unread, and is therefore unacceptable as the sole source of information. Ideally the patient information sheet should be:

- Short enough to read in a few minutes
- Easy to understand
- Available to take away (or keep a copy) as a record, for perusal at leisure and for discussion with friends and relatives.

Legal advisers to big organizations find it impossible to be brief, many doctors find it difficult to present the relevant information simply, and most doctors do not give the patient enough time and a copy to keep.

If the proposed study is a multicentre study organized by a big organization it may not be possible to modify the agreed patient information document. In this case an additional brief explanatory note from the local investigator, referring to the larger form, can be seen as a compromise.

When preparing your information sheet avoid long words and medical or scientific jargon. It is often helpful to show it to a lay person of modest intellect to find out if it makes sense to them. It is also important to studiously avoid coercive or authoritarian expressions. Do not say 'You will have to attend the surgery on three occasions . . .', but rather 'we will be asking you to . . .' or 'we would like you to . . .' or 'you will be invited . . .'.

Deciding how much information to give about drugs or procedures is quite difficult. In relation to a drug, for example, the patient will probably only want to know how extensively it has been used, whether it is safe and what effects it may have. A list of 38 rare adverse effects is inappropriate, but equally failure to mention that a drug causes serious headaches or bad indigestion in 5–10% of patients is inexcusable.

Most trials assess at least two alternative courses of action. Both treatments need to be explained, as do the terms randomization, single blind and double blind. The patient also needs to know if they may be on a placebo for any length of time.

Most ethics committees would like to see a sentence which says roughly 'if you do not wish to take part we will quite understand and will treat you in the normal way, which means . . .'. A second sentence may be helpful in some instances, to say 'if at any time you feel you do not wish to continue in the trial you can withdraw and there is no need to give any explanation'.

Four situations perhaps merit further comment:

The questionnaire. There is a belief that asking questions cannot be unethical and does not need a consent form. In fact, it may be unethical and it may be reasonable to require a consent form. In relation to questionnaires it is reasonable to ask:

- Will it be clear who is asking the questions and why?
- Could the questions be regarded as intrusive, too sexually explicit or irrelevant?
- Will any of the questions upset the patient? 'As you know, you are dying of cancer . . .'; 'Can you remember how you felt when your baby died . . .'.
- How long will it take to answer the questionnaire, and if it will take some time why should the person bother?
- In this, as in all forms of research, what steps will be taken to ensure confidentiality? Who may obtain access to the information, even if it is only the person's phone number, address or age?

The very ill and the dying. Clearly, extreme care is needed to avoid upsetting or overloading a patient. However, a patient with recurrent carcinoma of the ovary who has already had two courses of chemotherapy may want to try a new drug if it is available. This woman will know the situation. The information sheet can therefore begin with 'As you know we have been trying to control your cancer with drugs but the disease is not yet properly controlled . . .'. In addition, the document needs to warn about unpleasant side effects such as vomiting and hair loss.

The emergency situation. If the patient has just perforated an ulcer and is in severe pain and distress, this is not the time to have a detailed discussion about the complicated antibiotic regimens. In this situation it is probably better to persuade the ethics committee that both regimens are reasonable choices in the light of current knowledge, and that seeking consent would not be appropriate.

The patient who cannot give consent: Under this heading we should consider the unconscious patient, the young child and the mentally impaired. In these situations the investigator has to be particularly careful, and the LREC must see itself as having an even greater role as the patient's advocate, and the next of kin should be approached and asked to give consent. Particular care should be taken if the next of kin are in any way destabilized by the problems caused by looking after the relative.

The age of consent for children is being interpreted more liberally. In a legal sense a child may become an adult at 18, and in the past parents used to be solely responsible for giving consent on behalf of children under 16. It is now obvious that younger children may be able to understand quite clearly what may be involved in a particular project, and may have strong views on whether or not they wish to take part. This aspect has been investigated by two sixth-form students (Rylance, Bowen and Rylance 1995). It is now considered right to try to explain the study to the child if they are old enough to understand, to seek their approval, and only to override their wishes in exceptional circumstances, in which the child's decision could be clearly seen as detrimental to their long-term wellbeing.

LRECs – THE PROBLEMS

Difficulties may arise when the committee is slow or says no; when the committee is unsure; and when the investigator wants to perform a multicentre study.

LRECs are relatively autonomous and quite powerful. For the most part they are a group of individuals who give their time freely and work hard to be helpful and constructive. However, the increasing awareness of the need to obtain LREC approval has increased their workload. This may lead to delays which investigators may find unacceptable. Few researchers can be expected to wait more than a few weeks, and a committee which does not give an answer within eight weeks is being unethical because it encourages researchers not to bother to apply for approval.

Most committees will not say no without good reason: they usually ask questions or make suggestions if they feel that the application is not satisfactory. If they do not approve a project which the researcher is convinced is a good idea, then the first course of action is to carefully consider their reservations. The next step might be to seek the opportunity to explain your views face to face. Unfortunately, there is no defined appeal system.

The committee itself may suffer from lack of direction. There is no-one responsible for resolving ethical issues at a national level, although several authoritative bodies, including the Royal College of Physicians and the Department of Health, have provided some guidelines.

The greatest problem is that which faces the organization that wants to perform a multicentre trial. Unfortunately, each committee may reserve the right to comment on any study being performed in its area, and to require an application on its forms. Thus epidemiologists seeking to study a relatively uncommon problem may have to fill out large numbers of different forms and send them to a wide range of LRECs, which may have widely differing views on the one central protocol. This problem will have to be resolved by having some central committee which reviews the proposals, leaving the LRECs to comment briefly on the places and the people to be involved in their area.

CONCLUSIONS

Research ethics committees are there to protect and help both the patients and the researcher. Some of those contemplating performing a research project may consider putting together an application form for the LREC as an added burden. In fact, if you understand how the LREC works and what they want to know, it should not be difficult to write an application. Furthermore, the need to answer the questions posed by the committee usually encourages investigators to think more carefully and more clearly about what they want to do.

Further reading

Alberti, KGMM (1995) Local Research Ethics Committees. *BMJ.* **311**: 639–40.

Garfield P (1995) Gross district comparison of the applications to research ethics committees. *BMJ.* **311**: 660–1.

Pappworth MH (1967) *Human Guinea Pigs: Experimentation in Man.* Routledge and Kegan Paul, London.

Rylance G, Bowen C and Rylance J (1995) Measles and rubella vaccination – information and consent in children. *BMJ.* **311**: 923–4.

Thornton JG and Lilford RJ (1995) Clinical ethics committees. *BMJ.* **311**: 667–9.

While AE (1995) Ethics committees: impediments to research or guardians of ethical standards? *BMJ.* **311**: 661.

10

The role of the nurse in primary care research

Joyce Kenkre

INTRODUCTION

In 1994 a Department of Health (DoH) report to the NHS Central Research and Development Committee stated that 'a wide range of skills and methods will be needed to respond to the challenge of research at the interface between primary and secondary care'. One professional who was felt to be essential within the research team was the nurse. The role of the nurse within the primary care setting has developed greatly in the last ten years, with many now working in an extended role. In a study of practice nurses in 1991 only 15% had undergone research training, mainly within post-basic courses. However, 57% had been involved with research within their practice, reporting varying levels of involvement. For the Medical Research Council (MRC) study of mild hypertension 450 000 patients were screened, there were 16 000 trial participants, and this was undertaken by 1200 nurses nation-wide.

The importance of undertaking research is to find the answers to questions which will result in improved patient care. Traditionally, nurses have been taught to conduct certain procedures and not to question whether this is the best method or how that method was discovered or evolved. We therefore need to encourage questioning as part of our current practice. The motive for change should be the improvement of care. The Department of Health in its report 'Research for Health' stated that 'The objective of the NHS research and development strategy is to ensure that the content and delivery of care in the National Health Service is based on high quality research relevant to improving the health of the nation'. In this chapter it is proposed to discuss the possible future role of the nurse in research within primary care.

THE RESEARCH TEAM

The membership of the research team in primary care requires careful consideration. In any given project all members of the primary health care team have an important role to play. Prevalence studies may require the collection of information by receptionists, practice nurses, health visitors, midwives and general practitioners. The practice manager may undertake the role of coordinating the collection of information for his or her particular practice. It is important in any study requiring collection of information from a variety of health professionals, that all team members know who is involved and what their roles are. This may require a meeting to be arranged to inform all personnel about the protocol, procedures, timetable and documentation for the proposed study.

The nurse may undertake various roles, depending on the involvement she or he wishes to take, or the requirements of the study. Such roles may be:

- Project leader
- Project coordinator
- Design of the project
- Administration
- Patient care
- Interviewing patients
- Conducting diagnostic tests
- Support for the general practitioner
- Liaison with pharmaceutical companies.

This gives the nurse plenty of scope to develop and attain research skills in the primary care setting.

DATA COLLECTION

The role of the nurse in some research projects may be purely data collection for the general practitioner or the primary health care team, or for a larger regional or national study. This is a very important role, as the quality of the study will be reflected in the quality of the data collected. All personnel involved in the study should work in a standardized way with regard to the collection of data. This may necessitate a meeting between all the participants included in a research project to explain all aspects of the data collection.

Data should be collected systematically and documentation should be clear. Collection may be done manually or on computer file, and the data should be:

- As required by the research proposal
- Kept safely
- Recorded in the patient's notes
- The patient's confidentiality must be maintained.

PRIMARY SCREENING OF PATIENTS

Many studies stipulate inclusion and exclusion criteria for participation, to ensure that inappropriate patients are not entered into a study and therefore not inconvenienced or in anyway encouraged to take part in a study for which they are not eligible.

Screening the patients may include:

- Reviewing patient's notes
- Inviting them by letter to attend the surgery
- Checking the inclusion/exclusion criteria
- Informing the patient about all aspects of the study
- Ensuring patient consent is acquired prior to participation
- Taking patient's baseline assessments.

AUDIT

The DoH white paper *Working for Patients* defines medical audit as 'the systematic, critical analysis of the quality of medical care, including the procedures used for diagnosis and treatment, the use of resources, and the resulting outcome and quality of life for the patient'. Audit is increasingly being used within the primary care setting to assess what is actually happening in practice, so that change can occur. Unfortunately, audit is not popular; one reason for this may be that the initial collection of data may highlight weaknesses in the work performed by health professionals. However, the audit cycle can help in the improvement of quality of care for patients by:

- Defining criteria and standards
- Collecting data on performance
- Assessing performance against standards
- Identifying the need for change.

The audit cycle can also help all health professionals to develop a self-critical attitude to their own performance, and thereby maintain and improve the quality of care given to patients. In clinical practice time is, of course, at a premium, therefore there is an increasing necessity to justify that procedures undertaken are worth the time spent on them.

ACCOUNTABILITY

The United Kingdom Central Council for Nurses, Midwives and Health Visitors (UKCC) has set down a framework for nurses to assist them in exercising their accountability. In essence, accountability is part of professional practice, as a practitioner makes judgements in the care of patients and has to be accountable for those decisions. It is essential in research to maintain high standards, as future decisions may be made on the results found. Such decisions may involve national planning, or one practice or practitioner altering the care that they offer. This could have major implications if the results of the research are incorrect. Inaccuracies may be caused inadvertently by writing in a missing result in the study documentation, therefore giving false information. This compromises good research and poor standards are not acceptable.

In all aspects of research personnel should never:

- Record results that are untrue, especially if the reason is that the true reading was not in line with previous recordings
- Record a result if the test was not performed
- Forge another person's signature, even with their permission
- Perform tasks for which they have not received appropriate training.

It is important always to be able to feel when performing research tasks, that these are undertaken to the best of the person's ability and knowledge at the time. It has to be considered that clinical care may change in the light of new knowledge, so something examined in one way ten years ago may be out of vogue today.

RESERVATIONS

Many nurses have reservations about taking part in research, and few have none; the main one is lack of time. Another reason for reticence is lack of practical research skills: the theory may appear simple, but it is difficult knowing where to begin. This fear may be addressed by having a supporting role to begin with and developing skills through being part of a large project, or by joining a research group to gain experience and support.

Participating in research also raises the issue of the legal implications of trying new methods, devices or treatments in the routine care of patients. Health professionals want to improve care for their patients, hence the need for research. Therefore, when taking part in a study participants should feel that the research is worthwhile, that it is ethically correct and has gained the necessary approval, and that there is appropriate insurance coverage for patients and health professionals alike.

RESEARCH PROTOCOLS

If the nurse is going to be involved in a research project, either commissioned or otherwise, it is essential to read the study protocol and understand all components of the project. Ideally, the nurse may have had the opportunity to help develop the research protocol, thereby ensuring that all procedures can be undertaken within primary care. It is important that, if a research project is going to be conducted successfully in general practice, it can be organized in a practical manner within the setting, and that members of the primary health care team involved have been fully informed. Therefore, one should always:

- Read the research proposal thoroughly (may take several readings)
- Understand the methods to be used
- Make sure the research proposal can work in practice
- Check competence for tasks to be undertaken.

RESEARCH COORDINATOR

The research coordinator is the pivotal person in the organization of any large study, and therefore being able to communicate both in writing and verbally is a necessity. The coordinator has to ensure that all of the study data and procedures are recorded accurately and completely by everyone involved. There is also a need to work with other health professionals to develop an integrated approach.

The skills required are:

- Ability to organize
- Ability to work as a team member
- Ability to communicate
- Ability to motivate
- Ability to think ahead
- Self-discipline
- Computer literacy.

CLINICAL THERAPEUTIC TRIALS

Over recent years there has been a steady increase in the number of clinical therapeutic trials conducted in general practice. One of the reasons for this is that the patient with a disease that needs to be studied, without complications or other coexisting morbidity, is more likely to be found in general practice. A further reason is that drugs should be tested in the environment where they are most likely to be used. Trials have four phases, and the studies usually performed in general practice involve phases three and four. Some departments of general practice have specialized units that conduct phase two studies.

Phases of clinical therapeutic trials:

- *Phase one*. Systematic study of a product in human volunteers.
- *Phase two*. Randomized placebo-controlled trials to determine the efficacy and tolerability of the new compound for specific disease categories.
- *Phase three*. Randomized controlled trials comparing the study drug with established compounds, to confirm therapeutic effect and dose range. At this time studies are also undertaken to assess the effect on the elderly patient.
- *Phase four*. Post-marketing surveillance, which may include new therapeutic uses for the drug.

The role of the nurse in clinical therapeutic trials may vary between practices, and may also depend on the type of drug being tested. For some nurses their only involvement will be taking samples from the patient to be sent to a central laboratory, whereas in other practices the management of the study may be undertaken by the nurse, with the doctor only performing essential medical examinations. The nurse frequently completes the case report form (CRF), attends the investigator's meeting and liaises with the pharmaceutical company.

Possible tasks are:

- Taking vital sign assessments
- Taking samples for analysis
- Documenting results, including any side effects
- Administration of questionnaires (quality of life, activities of daily living)
- Administration of drugs
- Monitoring of protocol adherence
- Communicating in a multidisciplinary environment
- Communicating with pharmaceutical companies
- Arranging appointments
- Acting as the patient's advocate.

INFORMED CONSENT

In any study there is a continual debate on who should take informed consent, and whether it should be taken by a medical practitioner. In the new guidelines by the International Conference on Harmonization it has been set down that consent should be taken by the investigator. The investigator need not have a medical background, but there must be agreement for this and local research ethics committee approval. It is felt that nurses can explain research studies in a relaxed and non-intimidating way using language and terminology which is easily understood by the patient. It is important that the patient is not coerced into participating in a study, and time should be allowed for them to discuss their involvement in the study with their family. An information sheet should be given to the patient, containing details such as the purpose of the research, any investigative procedures, time commitment, risks and benefits to the patient, and a contact name and telephone number.

PATIENT'S ADVOCATE

As the patient's advocate the nurse's primary responsibility is to protect the patient's interests. This may cause a conflict of interest for the nurse, in that it may be a requirement of the research project that she does not fully inform the patient about a certain matter. For example, at the start of many studies there is a placebo baseline period when the patient at first takes placebo medication; it may create bias in the results if the nurse informs the patient of this. It is important for the investigator, who may be the general practitioner within the practice, that he or she can depend on the nurse to ensure strict adherence to the protocol, which has been approved by at least one ethics committee.

THE PRACTICE NURSE AND HIS OR HER OWN RESEARCH

Almost any aspect of a practice nurse's working day can provide a starting point for a research project. There is the opportunity to choose from such diverse activities as visiting patients in their home, running health promotion clinics in the surgery, to choosing what drugs/dressings to stock in the treatment room. Problems can be easily identified and questions asked. Many nurses prefer to research their area of particular expertise, so that their knowledge in their field of interest will increase. Whatever the reason for conducting a piece of research, it is important that it is a topic of interest to the individual and that the question is worth answering.

Points to consider for successful research

General:

- Keep research uncomplicated and to the point
- Research is not difficult, but think clearly and be organized
- People make research appear difficult, but usually the best research is simple
- Collaborate with other health care professionals
- Find assistance with administration
- Undertake research that can be completed and that gives a valid answer
- Make contact with other nurses with an interest in research
- Keep a positive attitude and enjoy the experience.

Specific:

- Develop a framework to answer the research question
- Choose a method suitable for the project
- Pilot the study
- Set out a systematic collection system for quality data
- Keep to a realistic number to enable you to answer the question
- If possible, talk to a statistician
- Publish your work.

PROMOTING RESEARCH

There is a need to develop quality nursing research within primary care. To achieve this a research culture has to be developed within the nursing profession. This may be a gradual process, which is likely to start by critically reading research and considering whether it may improve the way in which you practise. The next step may be to discuss research findings with colleagues, without feeling inhibited at the thought of putting forward a point of view. The more nurses discuss articles that they have read with one another and with colleagues from the whole primary care team, the more enjoyment and knowledge will be gained.

Unfortunately, nurses' experience of writing has largely been restricted to patients' notes, sometimes cryptically owing to lack of space. This is changing with the move to improve writing skills within post-basic courses. These courses are also providing a platform for gaining knowledge in research skills. There is a need for nurses to undertake their own research and to disseminate the findings. One way to achieve this is by publishing research findings, or by presenting them at a local meeting or nationally at conferences, although this may seem daunting. Support should be available within local practice nurse research groups, departments of general practice or departments of nursing. There is therefore a need to support nurses who are willing to promote research. There is also a need to get positive research findings into practice in the primary care setting, which will hopefully encourage others to develop these new skills.

Further reading

Barnes G (1981) The nurses' contribution to the Medical Research Council's Trial for mild hypertension. *Nursing Times.* **77**(29): 1240–1.

Bohaychuk W and Ball G (1993) *Standard Operating Procedures for Investigators*, 2nd edn. Good Clinical Research Practices, Hampshire.

Department of Health (1991) *Research for Health.* Department of Health, London.

Kenkre JE (1994) Research: is it for practice nurses? *Practice Nursing.* **5**(16): 39–40.

Kenkre JE (1994) Research: is research for practice nurses? *Practice Nursing.* **5**(17): 18–22.

R&D Priorities in Relation to the Interface Between Primary and Secondary Care. Report to the NHS Central Research and Development Committee (1994) Department of Health, London.

UKCC (1989) *Exercising Accountability.* UKCC, London.

Working for Patients (1989) Department of Health, London.

11

Systematic reviews and meta-analysis

Tim Lancaster

INTRODUCTION

Once an interesting question has been identified, the next step in planning a research project is to place the proposed project in the context of the existing evidence. The literature review is an obligatory part of study protocols, funding applications and papers which report the results of the research. Surprisingly little attention has, in the past, been given to methods for ensuring that reviews produce valid results, and there has been a growing recognition that the authors of many review articles do not report or use valid methods (Mulrow 1987). This failure to apply scientific principles to the synthesis of research is both wasteful and misleading. Inadequate reviews may lead to inappropriate clinical recommendations and to unnecessary duplication of research. For example, Antman *et al.* (1992) and Lau *et al.* (1992) showed that textbooks and review articles were failing to recommend treatments of proven value for myocardial infarction (most notably thrombolysis) many years after a careful summary of existing research would have shown their benefit. By the same token, treatments of no value (for example, lignocaine prophylaxis) continued to be recommended when there was strong evidence that they were ineffective.

Whether reviewing the literature to inform a research project, or preparing a review for publication, it is important to follow the same scientific principles that we apply to primary research. That is, reviews should address focused questions and should use explicit, reproducible methods. They should follow a formal, written protocol, and every effort should be made to reduce errors arising from bias and random error (the play of chance).

Reviews that follow such structured methods are called systematic reviews or overviews. Some systematic reviews may also use statistical techniques to combine data from different studies (meta-analysis). It is important that all researchers understand the principles of systematic reviews, not least because research proposals which do not include a valid summary of existing evidence will increasingly be rejected for funding. Traditional narrative review articles are already becoming difficult to publish. Indeed, performing a systematic review may be a very suitable first research project, since the principles of systematic reviews are really the principles of any good research method.

SETTING OBJECTIVES

The worst strategy in approaching a review is to set out to see 'what is there' without having any defined objectives. The most important first step therefore, is to formulate a clearly articulated question or hypothesis. In medical research, questions often concern an intervention (or exposure), a population and an outcome. Often the outcome of the intervention is measured in comparison with another intervention (or no intervention). This is a helpful way of structuring objectives.

For example, I was interested in the role of antiviral therapy for acute herpes zoster in general practice. Having thought about the clinical issues and discussed them with colleagues, I decided that the most important clinical issue was the effect on postherpetic neuralgia. So, the question became: 'In patients with acute herpes zoster (population), does treatment with antiviral chemotherapy (intervention) lead to a lower risk of persistent pain (outcome), compared to symptomatic treatment alone (comparison)?' (Lancaster et al. 1995). Having defined the research question in this way, it became much easier to construct a protocol to address it and to invite collaboration and comment from colleagues.

IDENTIFYING STUDIES

In research involving patients it is crucial that the subjects are identified in a way that does not lead to systematic bias. For example, the value of a particular clinical sign may be overestimated if it is studied in patients attending a hospital clinic and then applied to patients in general practice. The same is true of review articles, except that their subjects are studies rather than patients. Traditional review articles rarely state how the author searched for and identified the studies cited. This opens the process to bias. Authors may selectively cite studies which support their own prejudices, or rely on studies published in easily accessible journals.

In a systematic review there should be a clear description of the strategy used to identify studies, and this strategy should be as comprehensive as possible. As a minimum it should include a search of relevant electronic databases, such as MEDLINE, stating the search terms used. However, it is important to be aware of the limitations of electronic databases: not all relevant journals are indexed on MED-LINE. Even when studies are on MEDLINE, even the most sensitive search strategy will miss a significant proportion of relevant studies (usually because of the way they were indexed as they entered the database) (Adams *et al.* 1994; Dickersin *et al.* 1994). Other methods for identifying studies might include searching the reference lists of papers identified on MEDLINE, handsearching specialist journals, and consulting experts in the field. Valuable information may also be found in 'grey literature', for example as abstracts in conference proceedings, or may even be unpublished. Enlisting the help of a librarian can be invaluable in planning a search strategy.

Although there may not be resources to use all of the available methods, the most important principle is that there is a description of what was done, so that the reader can judge how reliable the search is likely to have been. For example, when searching for studies of treatments for herpes zoster we searched two electronic databases, scrutinized reference lists from previous reviews and textbooks, and wrote to specialists in the field and pharmaceutical companies involved in antiviral research. We documented this strategy in the final report.

CRITERIA FOR INCLUSION

Once the target population has been determined, the next step is to decide what kind of studies will be included. The criteria should specify both methodology and content (types of participants, interventions and outcomes). For example, in reviewing treatments for herpes zoster we decided that non-randomized studies would not offer sufficient bias control to provide reliable answers about whether treatment really worked. We therefore included only randomized controlled trials (methodology). Because we were interested in the use of antivirals in primary care, we excluded therapies that required intravenous administration or other hospital facilities (intervention). However, we judged that there was no good reason to assume that the treatments worked differently in specialist settings, so we included studies conducted both in primary care and in referral clinics, and included both ophthalmic and non-ophthalmic herpes zoster (participants). As our primary hypothesis was that treatment reduced the incidence of postherpetic neuralgia, we excluded studies that did not report data on pain at least one month after healing of the acute rash (outcome).

This example should not lead to the conclusion that the methods of the systematic review are only applicable to randomized trials. If our question related to a harmful exposure, then observational studies might be the most appropriate data source. For example, when considering the hypothesis that 'third-generation' oral contraceptives containing desogestrel or gestodene carry a greater risk of venous thrombosis in young women than 'second-generation' oral contraceptives, the main data source would be cohort and case control studies. Uncontrolled case series, however, would probably not be included in such a review.

DATA EXTRACTION

An important part of drawing up a review protocol involves the design of a reliable method for data extraction. Much time will be saved by careful development and piloting of a data extraction form. Not surprisingly, mistakes in data extraction are common, so it is helpful to have at least two individuals extract data and compare the results. Disagreements can be resolved by discussion, or by referral to a third party. It is important that the data extraction includes important descriptive data about the intervention and the participants, as well as the outcomes of interest. It is usually helpful to summarize descriptive data in tabular form in the final report. For example, in our herpes zoster review we abstracted data on the country of origin and funding sources, type and dose of treatment, nature of the control treatment, duration and completeness of follow-up, details of the randomization procedure and prevalence of pain at one, three and six months after treatment.

DATA SYNTHESIS

Having identified a set of studies which are the 'raw data' of the review article, some method must be used to synthesize their findings and draw conclusions. Authors of narrative review articles often do this qualitatively, that is, they discuss the findings of the different studies and draw some conclusion based on an intuitive sense of the overall direction of the evidence. Alternatively, they may use a semiquantitative method, where the number of positive studies is totted up, compared to the number of negative studies, and the winner takes all! Such methods are rather crude, and in particular may give inappropriate weight to smaller studies over larger ones. One solution is to perform meta-analysis, that is, to extract data from each of the studies and pool the results to give an overall estimate of, for example, treatment efficacy. The statistical techniques used in meta-analysis attach greater weight to larger studies than to smaller ones.

Going back to our herpes zoster example, we defined postherpetic pain as present or absent at the different time points. We then pooled data on this outcome measure from different studies to give an overall estimate of the likely effect of treatment, using a statistical method described by Yusuf and colleagues (1985). This allowed us to comment on how likely it was that the different treatments were effective.

Critics of meta-analysis often express the concern that such methods mix 'apples with oranges', and that it may be inappropriate to pool studies that have used different doses or studied different populations of patients. Clearly, judgement is important in deciding when it is sensible to perform meta-analysis. For example, in considering trials of acyclovir for herpes zoster, we produced separate estimates for studies that used high doses (> 4 g/day for 7–10 days) because of the suggestion that lower doses produced inadequate systemic levels of the drug. Within this dose range the studies appeared homogeneous – that is, variations in outcome were compatible with the play of chance alone, and pooling seemed to make sense. In considering trials of corticosteroids, on the other hand, the results reported ranged from large benefit to harm, and it seemed likely that the differences between trials were due to more than chance alone; therefore, combining them was probably not sensible.

Performing a meta-analysis may not be appropriate to all health care issues, and will be beyond the resources of many researchers. One solution may be to look for previous meta-analyses in the field and draw on these in reviewing research. In any case, the key principle remains: tell the reader what you did.

ASSESSING THE VALIDITY OF STUDIES

One of the most controversial areas in the science of reviewing research is how to assess the quality of the studies included. It seems almost self-evident that we should attach greater weight to well conducted studies than to those whose methodologies are more suspect. However, it has been surprisingly difficult to determine which quality criteria are important and how to apply them. In randomized trials, for example, the only criterion which has been empirically shown to affect outcome is the quality with which investigators attempt to blind participants to their treatment status (studies which do not report adequate randomization procedures tend to overestimate the likely benefits of treatment) (Schulz et al. 1995).

Part of the reason why the role of quality is not clear-cut is the problem of distinguishing what was done from what was reported. Studies may follow adequate procedures but not report them in sufficient detail to allow this to be judged. There are a number of possible ways of dealing with variations in quality. A threshold can be used, i.e. studies which do not meet certain agreed quality standards will be discarded altogether; quality scores can provide formal weighting in meta-analysis; or variations in quality can be used as a starting point for explaining differences between studies. For example, we found that the reported procedures in trials of corticosteroids for herpes zoster were of lower quality than those reported for acyclovir. This may explain the divergent effects of treatment reported in the different corticosteroid trials, and lead to caution in drawing conclusions about the value of this treatment.

Drawing conclusions

Few systematic reviews will produce such clear-cut results as in the example of treatments for myocardial infarction to which I referred in the introduction. Indeed, it may be rather disheartening when so much hard work does not lead to an unequivocal 'bottom line'. This was the situation we found ourselves in with our review of treatments for herpes zoster. Although there was no statistically significant effect of acyclovir on postherpetic neuralgia, we were unable to exclude the possibility that there may have been a modest benefit. This was because the number of patients studied in trials published at the time of the review, even when pooled between different studies, was insufficient to be certain that there was no effect of treatment. It is important that the conclusions of a review reflect this uncertainty, and accurately summarize the state of existing knowledge. This does not, of course, preclude making judgements and recommendations about what to do. For example, we suggested that, even without conclusive evidence, it was probably sensible to treat older patients with acyclovir since they are at higher risk of postherpetic neuralgia.

Keeping up to date

No matter how rigorously a review is conducted, its usefulness will rapidly decline as new research emerges. By the time our review of treatments for herpes zoster had been published, two important new studies had appeared. Much wasted effort could be avoided if those undertaking systematic reviews were to take responsibility for keeping them up to date and disseminating updated results. The Cochrane Collaboration, which was established in 1992, has exactly this goal, and aims to produce high-quality reviews which are regularly updated and disseminated in electronic format (Chalmers and Haynes 1994).

Further reading

Adams CE, Power A, Frederick K and Lefebvre C (1994) An investigation of the adequacy of MEDLINE searches for randomized controlled trials (RCTs) of the effects of mental health care. *Psychological Medicine.* **24**(3): 741–8.

Antman EM, Lau J, Kupelnick B, Mosteller F and Chalmers TC (1992) A comparison of results of meta-analyses of randomized control trials and recommendations of clinical experts. Treatments for myocardial infarction. *Journal of the American Medical Association.* **268**(2): 240–8.

Chalmers I and Haynes B (1994) Reporting, updating, and correcting systematic reviews of the effects of health care. *BMJ.* **309**: 862–5.

Dickersin K, Scherer R and Lefebvre C (1994) Identifying relevant studies for systematic reviews. *BMJ.* **309**: 1286–91.

Lancaster T, Silagy C and Gray S (1995) Primary care management of acute herpes zoster: systematic review of evidence from randomized controlled trials. *British Journal of General Practice.* **45**(390): 39–45.

Lau J, Antman EM, Jimenez Silva J, Kupelnick B, Mosteller F and Chalmers TC (1992) Cumulative meta-analysis of therapeutic trials for myocardial infarction. *New England Journal of Medicine.* **327**(4): 248–54.

Mulrow CD (1987) The medical review article: state of the science. *Annals of Internal Medicine.* **106**(3): 485–8.

Schulz KF, Chalmers I, Hayes RJ and Altman DG (1995) Empirical evidence of bias. Dimensions of methodological quality associated with estimates of treatment effects in controlled trials. *Journal of the American Medical Association.* **273**: 408–12.

Yusuf S, Peto R, Lewis J, Collins R and Sleight P (1985) Beta blockage during and after myocardial infarction: an overview of the randomized trials. *Progress in Cardiovascular Disease.* **27**(5): 335–71.

Additional reading

The most useful further source of information on this topic is contained in:
Chalmers I and Altman D (eds) (1995) *Systematic Reviews.* BMJ Publishing, London.

12

Critical appraisal of literature

Cathryn Thomas

INTRODUCTION

At first glance it may seem that the appraisal of other people's research has little to do with one's own, but being able to assess literature is essential for two reasons. First, to find out what has been done by others in the field in which you are interested. A literature review is the first stage of any research process. However, to read papers without attempting any appraisal of them is to miss the point. Topics may appear to have been covered but the context may be so different from your own, or the research methodology so flawed, that they do not inform the situation at all. The second reason for undertaking critical appraisal is to learn about research methodology. By systematically and rigorously appraising reports of research you will become familiar with different types of research and how different methods suit different questions. By reading the literature specific to your area of interest you will recognize particular methods that are suitable and commonly used, and may well recognize instruments (standard questionnaires or scales) which are particularly useful in the type of research you are contemplating.

The purpose of critical appraisal is to discover whether the methods and results of the research are sufficiently valid to produce useful information. It is not to assess the authors. Remember that the project may be the best that could be carried out, but because of unforeseen difficulties the results are of limited value.

When introducing people to the concept of critical appraisal for the first time I often find that they embrace it with an almost religious fervour; however, it is easy in that phase to become so obsessed with the *critical* part of it that every paper is found to be flawed. All research has shortcomings, and when one does one's own work – with the intention, of course, of producing the perfect study – one suddenly realizes just how difficult it is. In the sense in which it is used here, critical means being aware; not blindly believing things solely because they are in print; being systematic in one's analysis; and applying standards.

METHOD FOR QUANTITATIVE STUDIES

There are many ways of appraising written work: this is one. Sackett *et al.*'s book *Clinical Epidemiology. A Basic Science for Clinical Medicine*, and the more recent and somewhat simpler JAMA's *User's Guides to the Medical Literature* probably give the definitive method, but this chapter pulls together their ideas and those of other authors into a (fairly) concise form. Highly recommended is *Critical Reading for Primary Care*, edited by Roger Jones and Ann-Louise Kinmonth.

Remember that there are different types of reading. One quickly scans the titles to have a sense of whether one wants to read on; one might then browse through the abstract to get a feel of whether a paper is worth reading, and then one might read it.

At the scanning point one is filtering out the papers that are of no interest. Next one needs to look at the abstract. Just by reading it through you should be able to tell whether the paper is worth looking at critically. If it has nothing to offer your clinical practice, or is unbelievable, you may choose to turn to something else. Obviously there are times when you have no choice but to continue. At this stage also one will hopefully be able to identify the fatally flawed paper. This is one where there is such a gross problem that it makes it pointless to read on. The authors might, for example, have lost 50% of their patients on follow-up (it is, of course, unlikely that such a paper would get published, but some fatally flawed papers do).

Assuming that one has decided to read the paper, this is one way of doing it. You will develop your own method as you go along, but this chapter should help you at the start.

- *First*, skim the whole paper. Do not concentrate on detail at this stage. Try to get a feel of what the paper is about and whether it makes sense. By the time you have read the paper through once you should be able to answer three questions:

  1. What is the message?

  2. Do I believe it?

  3. If true, how does it affect what I do at present?

- *Second*, read it through carefully, noting significant points, e.g. for quantitative studies: hypothesis, number of subjects, significant results, discussion points etc.

as you go along. For qualitative studies: description of the participants, range of opinions expressed etc. Write them down, creating your own summary.
- *Finally*, go through the whole paper systematically using the suggestions that follow to look at each section in detail.

Do not be tempted to miss out the first stage. Common sense is important. It is possible for an important paper to be apparently full of flaws but still be of fundamental importance because it contains or raises an idea not dealt with effectively anywhere else. One can become so bogged down in detail that one cannot see the wood for the trees.

Review of the abstract

The *BMJ* now uses structured abstracts. These comprise:

- Objectives
- Design
- Setting
- Subjects
- Main outcome measures
- Results
- Conclusion.

Other journals do not necessarily use this system, but their abstracts should contain all this information.

Serious flaws can be identified at this stage (the fatally flawed paper). Is the summary a true reflection of what the rest of the paper states?

Who are the authors? Studies which are about general practice but have no GP input are generally less credible than those by GPs.

Is the journal peer refereed? This means do they send submissions to reviewers or do they just accept any copy that is sent to them?

The JAMA's *User's Guides* ask three questions of a paper:

- Are the results valid?
- What are the results?
- Will the results help me in patient care?

Different types of questions are answered by different methods of research, and different points should be looked for when appraising them. For example, a study looking at a new drug should use a randomized controlled trial, and one needs to ask questions about 'blinding', whereas a study looking at prognosis would use a cohort study, and one would be concerned with the study being of sufficient length and completeness. What follows attempts to ask general questions rather than specific ones. For specific questions look at the JAMA's *User's Guides*.

Introduction

Objectives

What are the objectives of the study or the questions to be answered?

Are they clearly stated (unambiguous)?

Is there a hypothesis?

If so, can you identify the hypothesis easily? If not, why not?

If there is no hypothesis is this appropriate?

Is the study ethical? Has an ethical committee approved it?

Literature review

As far as you can tell, is this adequate?

Is it informative?

Method

Design

What type of study is it? (Box 12.1)

Is the design appropriate to the objectives?

If a questionnaire is used, was it piloted before use in the study?

Does it seem to have been well designed?

If interviews are used, have the interviewers been adequately trained?

Have efforts been made to standardize the interviews?

Is there a control group or standard of comparison?

What is the source of the controls?

Is matching applicable?

If so, is it adequate?

What entry and exclusion criteria are used?

Are they valid?

Is the timespan appropriate? The time allowed must be long enough for the outcome to occur.

Box 12.1 Study design

This should be stated in the abstract and at the beginning of the methods section. Most studies fall into the categories below. Many are combinations of these.

- *Case report*: A description of one interesting and unusual case.
- *Case series*: A description of several cases in which no attempt is made to answer specific hypotheses or to compare results with another group of cases.
- *Cross-sectional study*: A survey of the frequency of disease, risk factors or other characteristics in a defined population at one particular time.
- *Cohort study*: An observational study of a group of people with a specified characteristic or disease who are followed up over a period of time to detect new events. Comparisons may be made with a control group. Interventions are not normally applied.
- *Control study*: An observational study in which characteristics of people with a disease (cases) are compared with those of selected people without the disease (controls).
- *Controlled trial*: An experimental study in which an intervention is applied to one group of people and the outcome compared with that in a similar group (controls) not receiving the intervention.

Setting

Where does the study take place?

Is the setting appropriate for the study? 'General practice' studies lose credibility when they use patients in hospital outpatient clinics.

Can you relate the findings to where you work?

Subjects

Who is being studied?

Is the whole population being studied or has a sample been taken?

If there is a sample, how was it selected – randomly or non-randomly?

Is there selection bias, i.e. have their sources of selection made the sample atypical or unrepresentative of the population being studied? (see Box 12.2)

If there is bias, how have they dealt with it? Biases may not be able to be eliminated, but efforts should be made to minimize them.

Was the sample big enough? To answer this question properly requires a knowledge of factors which you may not have at your fingertips (e.g. size of the standard error).

We are more concerned here with whether the sample size is too small to be representative.

Were all the patients entered in the study accounted for at the end?

Outcome measures

Are there clear definitions of the terms used, e.g. diagnostic criteria, measurements made and outcome criteria?

What are the criteria?

How were they developed?

Are they clinically relevant and relevant to the objectives?

Are they reliable and reproducible?

Would all doctors accept this end-point?

Were they consistent for all the subjects?

Are there possible biases in measurement, e.g. deaths, drop outs, missing data, and if so what was done to deal with them?

Has observer bias been removed or minimized?

Results

Are the findings clearly and objectively presented?

Is there sufficient detail for the reader to judge for him or herself?

Was the response rate adequate? (should ideally be > 70%).

Are the results internally consistent, i.e. do they add up to the right numbers?

How many non-responders or lost to follow-ups are there?

What happens to non-responders? (It should be assumed that a worst-case scenario applies, and they should be put in the treatment failure group. This is known as 'intention to treat'.)

Are the data worthy of statistical analysis? If so, are the methods used appropriate to the nature and source of the data?

Is the analysis correctly performed and interpreted?

Are there sufficient data and analysis to tell whether 'significant differences' may in fact be due to a lack of comparability between groups, e.g. in terms of age, sex or clinical characteristics?

Box 12.2 Biases

- *Extraneous treatments:* In controlled trials subjects are exposed to treatments in addition to the one being evaluated. These need to be identified and the results interpreted.
- *Contamination:* In controlled trials one group is affected by another, e.g. one group tells the other about changes in diet.
- *Changes of time:* Data collected from two groups at different times. Differences may be due to the measurement over time, not to a real difference between the groups.
- *Confounding factors:* Distorting influences may exist in studies examining the association between a risk factor and disease, where the purpose is to find out whether the association is real or spurious (caused by a confounding factor influencing both the risk factor and the disease). In such studies it is necessary to account for possible confounding factors. This may be satisfied by matching in the selection of controls, or by evidence of comparability between cases and controls. Age and sex are frequent confounding factors.

Have any outside factors which could have influenced the results been taken into account?

Discussion

Have the initial objectives been reached?

Is the question answered, the hypothesis proved or disproved?

Have the data been interpreted objectively?

Are the conclusions justified by the results?

Which are not?

Are the conclusions relevant to the original question?

Are any results not discussed?

Is there an explanation for this?

Are the results clinically significant?

Are they relevant to you and your practice, and/or to general practice as a whole?

Ask three questions:

1. *Bias:* Are the results biased in a certain direction? This may not necessarily negate the value of the study as long as the direction and magnitude of the bias

are known and are recognized by the researchers. Problems start when they fail to recognize bias or fail to discuss it.

2. *Confounding*. Are there any serious confounding or other distorting influences? Often these cannot be adequately accounted for in the analysis, and may have a substantial effect on the results.

3. *Chance*. Is it likely that the results occurred by chance? The answer depends primarily on the statistics, and help from a statistician may be needed.

METHOD FOR QUALITATIVE STUDIES

As much rigour needs to be applied to reading qualitative work as quantitative.

Abstract

Is the area being investigated of importance and of interest to you? Have they picked the right methodology, i.e. should this be a qualitative study? Do they have a clear research question? Qualitative research is inductive rather than deductive in nature, that is, the research informs the question, but by the time the research is written up the question should be clear. Is the context of the research clear?

Introduction

This is as for a quantitative study.

Method

Generally much more space is taken to explain the method of qualitative research. The methods cannot be written in the 'shorthand' of quantitative research and, to be explicit about the methods used and to make clear the rigour of what has been done, qualitative researchers should go into detail.

When choosing subjects for a qualitative study the researcher may not necessarily be looking for a random sample, and it is certainly not necessary to achieve statistical representativeness. Samples may be chosen at random or may not. Subjects with some particular characteristic that is being studied are selected, and within that sample a range of ages, both genders and a spread of other factors will be sought. The researcher should be aiming for a sample that is sufficiently comprehensive to allow generalizability. Bad sampling is where the subjects are chosen purely because they are available.

For those used to reading quantitative papers the issue of generalizability is one they find difficult to understand. How can an interview study of 40 people be generalized? This is to miss the point somewhat. Qualitative researchers do not say 'what I have found applies to the whole world' (nor would most quantitative researchers, of course): they are, by virtue of their detailed descriptions, giving you the opportunity to have an insight into the views of their subjects. If their subjects are like your patients, or not so different that they are from another population entirely, then you will be able to draw conclusions from the research. The issue here is not so much generalizability as transferability. Can the results be transferred to your patients who are like those studied?

The detail given in the method should include a justification of why the particular method of data analysis was chosen and how it was undertaken. The themes and concepts emanating from the research should be clearly identified. The analysis should be repeated by at least one other researcher to ensure reliability. Sometimes it is appropriate for quantitative techniques to be used to test the qualitative conclusions, but this is not always the case.

Results

Again, the results section is likely to be longer than for a quantitative paper. Enough of the original evidence, e.g. transcript quotations, should be given (clearly identified using a code) to satisfy the reader that the interpretation of the evidence is fair. The authors should also give evidence that they have sought observations that would have contradicted or modified the analysis – so-called disconfirming evidence.

Conclusions

The conclusions should be based upon the evidence presented and its analysis. The nature of qualitative research is inductive, i.e. it leads to a question rather than from one, and this may be the final conclusion.

Box 12.3 Some useful definitions

- **Validity** The extent to which measurements reflect the true situation.
- **Reliability or reproducibility** The extent to which the same results would have been obtained if the measurements had been taken by a different observer on a different day.
- **Sensitivity** The measure of a test's ability to detect x, i.e. true positive (where x is the variable being tested).
- **Specificity** The measure of a test's ability to correctly identify the absence of x, i.e. true negative (where x is the variable being tested).
- **Study sample** The group selected to participate. For the research to be applicable and relevant to other populations, this group must be representative of the study population.

- **Study population** The group from which the study sample is drawn. This should be typical of the target population.
- **Target population** The wider population to whom the research might apply.
- **Incidence** New events occurring in a defined population within a specified time.
- **Prevalence** The number of cases of a disease or condition which exist in a defined population in a designated period of time.
- **Bias** A form of systematic error, leading to consistent over- or underrecording of the true situation. It cannot be reduced by increasing the size of the sample and its effect is difficult to quantify. It must be recognized and removed.
- **Random error** Error that occurs by chance. It leads to a less precise estimate of whatever is being measured, but the degree of imprecision can be statistically estimated and the effect can be offset by making the study larger.

Further reading

Britten N, Jones R, Murphy E and Stacy R (1995) Qualitative research methods in general practice and primary care. *Family Practice.* **12**(1): 104–14.

JAMA *User's Guides to the Medical Literature*

JAMA 1993; **270**: 2598–601

JAMA 1994; **271**: 59–63

JAMA 1994; **271**: 389–91

JAMA 1994; **271**: 703–7

JAMA 1994; **271**: 1615–19

JAMA 1994; **272**: 234–7

JAMA 1994; **272**: 1367–71

JAMA 1995; **273**: 1292–5

JAMA 1995; **273**: 1610–13

Jones R and Kinmonth A-L (eds) (1995) *Critical Reading for Primary Care.* Oxford University Press, Oxford.

Mays N and Pope C (eds) (1996) *Qualitative Research in Health Care.* BMJ, London.

Sackett DL, Haynes RB, Guyatt GH and Tugwell P (1991) *Clinical Epidemiology. A Basic Science for Clinical Medicine*, 2nd edn. Little, Brown and Company, Boston.

Silman AJ (1995) *Epidemiological Studies: a Practical Guide.* Cambridge University Press, Cambridge.

13

Mastering MEDLINE and managing references

Andy Wearn and David Rogers

This chapter aims to address the following questions:

- Why is a literature review important?
- What medical reference sources exist?
- How do I search the literature using an electronic database? The MEDLINE service is used as an example. The chapter will familiarize you with the service and guide you through practical searching
- How can I store and use references on a subject? Includes electronic reference management packages.

This chapter will give you a basic theoretical understanding of these subjects. The next step should be to gain 'hands-on' experience. Most medical libraries offer training sessions which will allow you to see how it all works in practice.

INTRODUCTION

Before putting up a tent you have to assess the site. Is the ground suitable for pegging out? How exposed is the site? If the ground is rough and uneven, is there a niche for your tent? Who else is camping there? If its hard to find a patch of ground then you probably ought to move on to another site.

We make no apologies for concocting this analogy, but will attempt to put it into context. Once you have a research idea the next step is a literature review. This is a vital step in the research process for a number of reasons:

- At its simplest, a search lets you see what has already been published within the area of interest
- Previous studies might highlight difficult and unfruitful research areas within the subject chosen
- You may be able to identify a new angle or niche
- Other studies may suggest a methodology which you had not considered
- Often it results in the evolution of your research question or hypothesis
- If there is already a comprehensive literature on your chosen subject, you might want to think again
- You may identify a useful research tool or scale
- If certain authors' names crop up regularly, it is sometimes beneficial to make contact
- Most importantly, it gives you a background and context to the proposed research and prevents you from reinventing the wheel.

Good ideas need to be supported by a good literature search.

The body of medical and social science literature is enormous and is added to continuously. Sifting through it might at first seem very daunting, but help is at hand.

MEDICAL REFERENCE SOURCES

Some readers will have already used *Index Medicus* or had experience of searching medical databases such as MEDLINE and BIDS to find references. For the uninitiated or the novice user, MEDLINE and BIDS are electronic databases stored on a central mainframe computer or on CD-ROM disks (updated monthly). Using a personal computer (PC) and appropriate software the database can be interrogated to identify references on particular subject areas. Most commonly this is done on a dedicated PC in a library which subscribes to the service.

Access to databases

You will find that all medical school libraries and most postgraduate centre libraries have this facility, and the service may be provided free or at a charge. Usually you have to book a timed session for searches. At some postgraduate centres a member of staff will perform the search for you. However, it is far better to do this yourself as the search is a dynamic process and will usually involve decisions which the enquirer is best placed to make. A third-party search may produce results which are too broad or have strayed from their objective.

Index Medicus is also found in medical libraries. This predates the information technology revolution and is the paper equivalent of MEDLINE. Using it is cumbersome, desperately slow and frustrating compared with the electronic equivalents.

An alternative for those who have a PC at home or at work is to access a database remotely. This is referred to as 'online' searching. To do this you need a PC with Windows or Apple Mac, a modem, a standard phoneline plug-in point and a distant service provider. In simple terms, you then call up the provider from your PC and search the database remotely. If you are a member of the BMA then they provide a free service, although of course you pay for the connecting phone call (see also Chapter 15). The main drawback is that it is well used and there is a limit to the number of users at any one time. Therefore, you may have to try several times to gain access, or choose 'quieter' times of day (or night). Table 13.1 gives some examples of electronic databases.

BIDS is the Bath Information and Data Services and gives access to ISI & EMBASE.

MEDLINE is the most common service available and has therefore been chosen as a practical example. Other electronic databases are similar in their syntax and behaviour, so the basic skills and commands are largely transferable.

Table 13.1 Examples of electronic databases

Database	Main topics	Contains references since	Online	CD-ROM
MEDLINE	All of medicine (including dentistry & veterinary medicine)	1966	Yes	Yes
ISI	Consists of four databases each covering specific areas: Science Citation Index, Social Sciences Citation Index, Arts & Humanities Citation Index and Index to Scientific & Technical Proceedings	1982	Yes	No
CANCERLIT	Cancer & epidemiology	1963	Yes	Yes
ASSIA	Sociology, psychology, cultural anthropology, politics & economics	1987	Yes	Yes
CINHAL	Nursing & paramedical disciplines	1983	Yes	Yes
EMBASE	Focus on therapeutics & pharmacology	1974	Yes	Yes
DHSS-DATA	Health service, administration & management	1983	Yes	No

MEDLINE

MEDLINE is a huge international database of biomedical and associated health literature compiled by the National Library of Medicine (NLM) in the United States. It has a wide coverage, indexing around 3600 journals in every major world language from 70 countries.

It is so popular that first-time researchers may easily assume that a MEDLINE search will have covered the whole subject; unfortunately, this is not the case, as MEDLINE's coverage, although extensive, is not absolutely comprehensive.

It has a strong US bias, which excludes some important UK journals such as the *British Journal of Family Planning*, as well as some prominent foreign-language titles. Its coverage of UK health administration and management is patchy, likewise for the professions allied to medicine, such as physiotherapy and occupational therapy.

Other databases, notably DHSS-DATA for management material, and The Cumulative Index of Nursing and Allied Health Literature (CINAHL) for paramedical topics, may have to be cross-referenced to improve retrieval. MEDLINE is an excellent and obvious starting point for literature searching, but do consult your local librarian for advice, particularly if potentially costly online searching is involved.

Box 13.1 MEDLINE
- MEDLINE is often the best, although not the only place to begin your search
- MEDLINE's coverage is not all-inclusive: you may need to consider other databases
- Ask your librarian for help and advice

Getting started: the basics

It is assumed that the reader is familiar with using a PC. MEDLINE is offered under licence by a number of suppliers (e.g. OVID and Silver Platter). Both DOS and Windows versions of the search engines are produced, which simply affects how the screen looks and, to some extent, the speed. Most systems carry reference data since 1990 or 1992. Some CD-ROM systems and the mainframe will have earlier references; if this is the case then you can choose a different year band in which to search. **This guide is based on OVID-MEDLINE and the screenshots are from the Windows version.**

The initial screen you are presented with has a command line box, output display box and command menu system that is similar to every other PC application you have seen. Commands are selected from menus and text is added at the prompt (as you get more experienced, commands can be entered as freehand text).

- When you are ready the system performs a search and lets you know how many references on the subject it has found; these are known as 'hits'.
- A group of hits is called a set.
- Each search, manipulation of a previous set of hits, or refinement is listed numerically on the output screen.
- At any time you can view the references in a chosen set. When you select this function you are able to choose the detail with which it is viewed (from title only to the whole record held, usually including an abstract).

- Selected references can be printed or downloaded to a floppy disk.
- A Help screen is available from the menu or function key F1.

There are two main approaches to searching MEDLINE: MeSH searching and text-word searching.

MeSH – medical subject headings

'The key to effective MEDLINE searching'

This is the controlled vocabulary or thesaurus used by the NLM to index journal articles for MEDLINE. MeSH is arranged alphabetically (with cross-references). It is also viewable as a classified structure or 'tree', in which related terms are shown in proximity to each other and in their relationship with broader and narrower subjects. The 'tree' is also available via the 'Tools' option and will prompt for a known MeSH term, which will then be displayed in its place in the hierarchy. The idea is similar to other classification systems, the most familiar of which will be the Dewey system found in public libraries.

At the initial screen the default prompt is for a MeSH term search. In other licensees' version you may have to choose MeSH term searching from the 'Tools' option on the top command line (called the 'Thesaurus' in some versions).

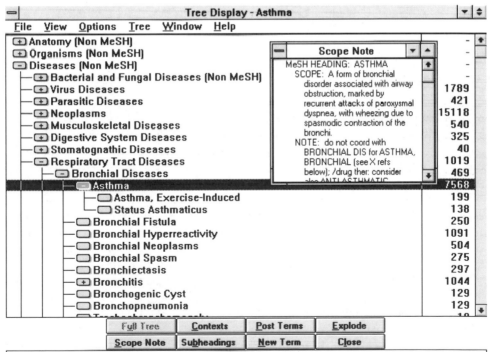

Figure 13.1 Screenshot: The 'tree'.

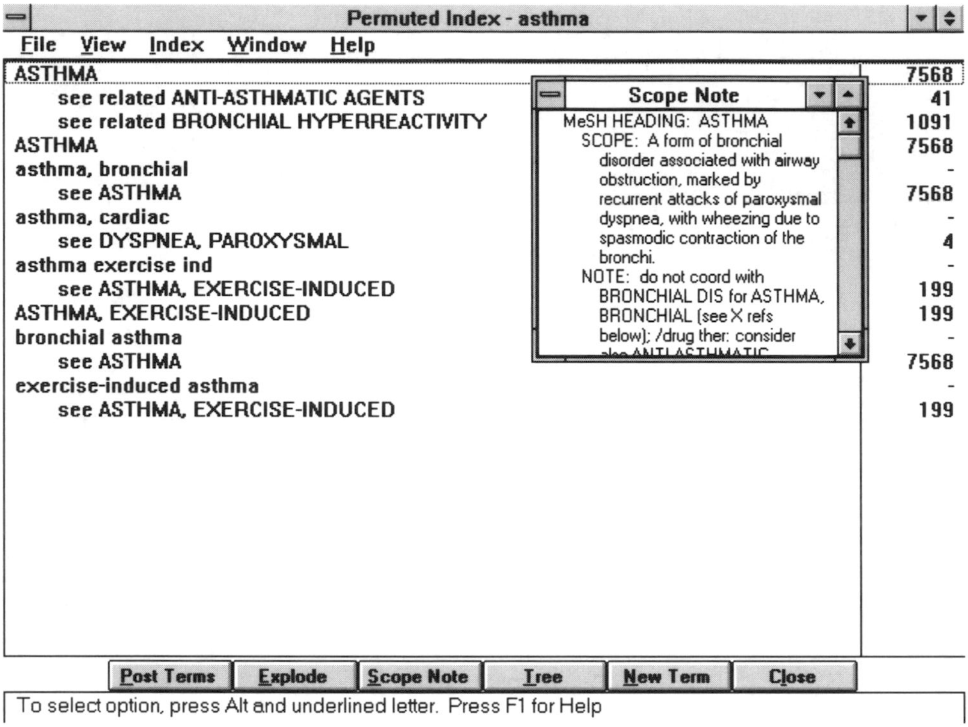

─	Permuted Index - asthma	▼ ♦

File   View   Index   Window   Help

ASTHMA		7568
see related ANTI-ASTHMATIC AGENTS	─ **Scope Note** ▼ ▲	41
see related BRONCHIAL HYPERREACTIVITY	MeSH HEADING: ASTHMA ♦	1091
ASTHMA	SCOPE: A form of bronchial	7568
asthma, bronchial	disorder associated with airway	-
see ASTHMA	obstruction, marked by recurrent attacks of paroxysmal	7568
asthma, cardiac	dyspnea, with wheezing due to	-
see DYSPNEA, PAROXYSMAL	spasmodic contraction of the	4
asthma exercise ind	bronchi.	-
see ASTHMA, EXERCISE-INDUCED	NOTE: do not coord with BRONCHIAL DIS for ASTHMA,	199
ASTHMA, EXERCISE-INDUCED	BRONCHIAL (see X refs	199
bronchial asthma	below); /drug ther: consider	-
see ASTHMA	also ANTI ASTHMATIC ♦	7568
exercise-induced asthma		-
see ASTHMA, EXERCISE-INDUCED		199

Post Terms	Explode	Scope Note	Tree	New Term	Close

To select option, press Alt and underlined letter. Press F1 for Help

Figure 13.2 Screenshot: The 'permuted index'.

Other options in the 'Tools' menu are 'Permuted index', 'Scope' and 'Tree'. Choosing 'Permuted index' will prompt for a single word, e.g. ASTHMA, and will go directly to that term in the alphabetical listing, showing the number of occurrences of the term on the right of the screen. Also shown will be the preferred forms for other variations of the term, e.g. asthma, cardiac see DYSPNEA, PAROXYSMAL.

In Windows versions a dialogue box will also be displayed in a pop-up window, explaining the meaning of the term and any related headings you may also want to consider searching under (in DOS versions choose 'Scope' from the 'Tools' menu). Clicking on a term, followed by 'Post terms' and then 'Close', will return you to the main search window and display the number of hits for that term.

It is important to remember that American spelling and terminology is used throughout MeSH, so that entering BREAST CANCER for a Tree search will cause an error message to be displayed stating TERM NOT FOUND. Entering FOETUS will result in a similar electronic shrug of the shoulders, whereas BREAST NEOPLASMS and FETUS bring instant success. More importantly for primary care research, GENERAL PRACTICE is coded as FAMILY MEDICINE or FAMILY PRACTICE.

How to refine the search

'All documents'/'Restrict to focus'

Indexing is carried out in such depth that MeSH headings are assigned to papers even when the subject is only touched upon. If a single term is being searched, it may be advantageous to 'Restrict to focus'. This selects only papers where the heading is the main theme.

Subheadings

These allow a search to be more focused still. Only those headings specific to your chosen term will be offered, e.g. DIET THERAPY would not appear as a subheading for FRACTURES. Any number of valid subheadings may be selected.

Although this may take some getting used to, the advantage of using MeSH headings is that all alternative spellings, abbreviations, acronyms and synonyms are covered automatically, which is not the case in textword searching.

You may have heard that up to 40% of potential 'hits' from a MEDLINE search may go unretrieved. This may be due to inconsistent indexing by the NLM, an unsophisticated approach to searching on the part of the user, or a combination of the two. Practice will certainly improve your searching technique.

Textword (freetext) searching

This can be very effective and is sometimes the only option for your particular subject. This will be for times when no MeSH heading exists, the MeSH terms are inadequate or you wish to search specifically for a particular phrase. Textword searching may also be useful in conjunction with MeSH searching or to identify the best MeSH terms to use in a search strategy. Simply enter the text and it will be searched for exactly as typed, in the records on the database.

This is particularly good when searching for medical syndromes, as these are usually known by several synonyms and the rarer ones often have no MeSH heading assigned to them. Furthermore, MeSH terminology is constantly changing, and it sometimes pays to use textword searching to help identify relevant references published before the introduction of a suitable MeSH heading.

A good example of this is the MeSH heading ANGELMAN SYNDROME, introduced in 1993. A textword search for HAPPY PUPPET (a synonym for Angelman's) will retrieve relevant papers that have not been assigned ANGELMAN SYNDROME as a MeSH heading, or MOVEMENT DISORDERS, the pre-1993 heading.

This demonstrates that even in a highly accurate database environment such as MEDLINE, mistakes in indexing can slip through, so textword searching can be used as an additional 'belt and braces' approach.

The main drawback with textword searching is that, to be fully effective, it needs to include all possible alternative spellings, synonyms, acronyms and abbreviations, as only the characters entered will be searched for, and only in the title and abstract fields (except in the OVID Full Text Collection, in which the whole paper is indexed).

Nurses in particular will know that titles of papers in, for example, *Nursing Times*, often give no clue as to the subject content, and so are not much help in textword searching. Another frequently encountered problem is that of 'false drops', or retrieving irrelevant material that happens to contain an occurrence of the chosen textword in a different context.

Truncation

The $ sign may be used to perform 'right-hand truncation'. Adding the $ sign to the end of a word means that the database will search for the word chosen plus all occurrences with different endings. e.g. POISON$ would retrieve POISON, POISONS and POISONING, as well as POISONER, POISONERS and POISONINGS. This can therefore be a frustrating source of 'false drops' if not used with care.

Box 13.2 Searching MEDLINE
- Use textword searching where no suitable MeSH term exists, or to assist in choosing one (by retrieving a relevant paper by keyword and checking the MeSH terms assigned to it)
- Choose textwords and/or truncation with care to avoid false drops
- Also use textword searches to supplement and cross-reference with MeSH searching
- In most cases searching on MeSH headings will give better results

---

Returning to our earlier example of the term ASTHMA, the mapping process may involve the following steps:

- Mapping of a word or phrase to the appropriate MeSH heading
- Selection of broader/narrower terms, or 'exploding'
- 'Restricting to focus'
- Application of subheadings, e.g. DRUG THERAPY.

What then appears on the screen is:

exp *asthma/dt

The **exp** shows that the term which follows has been 'exploded'; the preceding **asterisk** that 'Restrict to focus' has been chosen; and the **dt** that the subheading 'drug therapy' has been applied.

Once this shorthand becomes familiar, after a little practice, the prompts of the mapping system can be bypassed in favour of entering expressions directly into the search box, thus opening the way to faster and more efficient searching.

Further refining your search

Even after going through the stages of mapping, you may still be faced with an impossibly large set which needs further refining. It is now that the various Limit commands come into play. The Limit option on the top command line displays those you may use most often. Choosing any of these (other than 'All limits') will apply to your last search set. If you want to limit a previous set, use 'Limit set' on the bottom command line.

'Local holdings' may be useful if you need immediate access to original articles, as only journals held in the host library will be retrieved.

If the library also subscribes to the new OVID Full Text Collection, a 'Full text' option will be displayed, enabling access to the full text and graphics of the 15 titles (e.g. *BMJ* and *Lancet*) currently included.

'Human' will exclude animal studies if they are a feature of your chosen term, as in the various neoplasm headings.

'English language' obviously excludes foreign-language papers, but bear in mind that many of these may carry an English abstract.

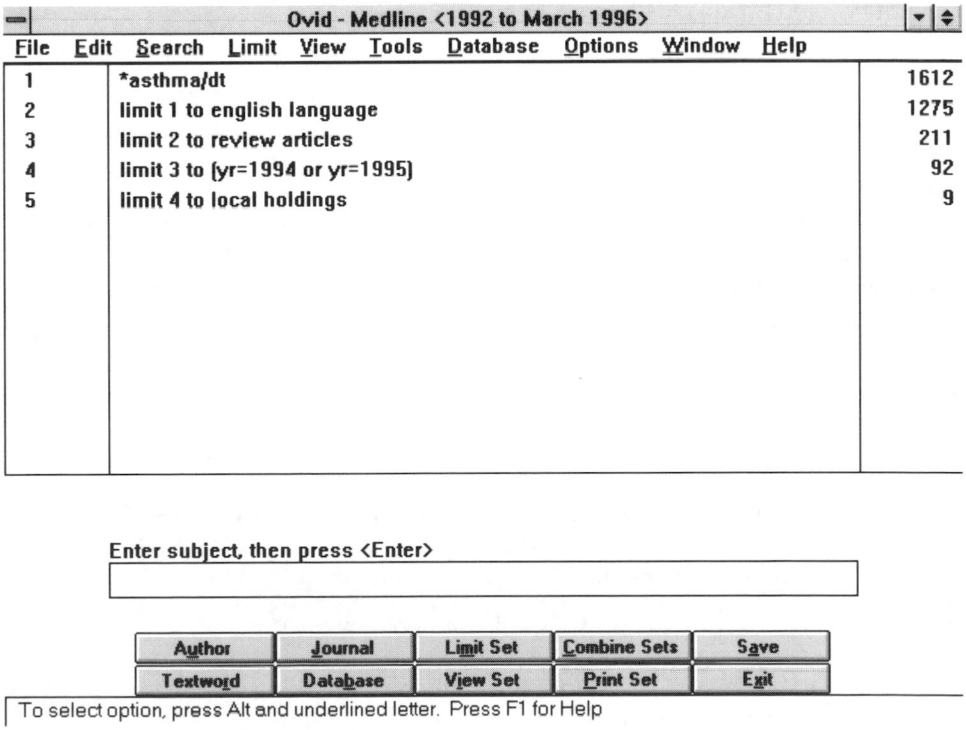

Ovid - Medline <1992 to March 1996>	
File Edit Search Limit View Tools Database Options Window Help	
1 *asthma/dt	1612
2 limit 1 to english language	1275
3 limit 2 to review articles	211
4 limit 3 to [yr=1994 or yr=1995]	92
5 limit 4 to local holdings	9

Enter subject, then press <Enter>

Author	Journal	Limit Set	Combine Sets	Save
Textword	Database	View Set	Print Set	Exit

To select option, press Alt and underlined letter. Press F1 for Help

Figure 13.3 Screenshot: Refining the search.

'Review articles' are ideal for a quick overview of a subject, and often have large numbers of useful references appended.

'Abstracts' mainly excludes correspondence, but use with care as editorials will also be omitted. Over 60% of MEDLINE records after 1975 include an author's abstract. Databases which offer independently written abstracts (for example Excerpta Medica) are invariably much more expensive to produce and are therefore less popular with libraries.

'All limits' in effect gives access to the 'Limit set' command on the bottom line and features several useful options.

'Latest update' (available only on the CD-ROM versions of MEDLINE, which are updated monthly) allows the facility to use saved search strategies, combined with this limit to create regular updates.

'AIM journals' limits the search to the 119 core clinical journals which form the Abridged Index Medicus collection. These are the ones most likely to be found in small to medium-sized medical libraries.

'Age groups' is confined to humans, so it is unnecessary to also limit to 'Human' when using this option. If a range of ages is required, it is possible to 'explode' the heading CHILD to cover birth to age 18, and similarly ADULT to include ages 19 and above.

'Publication types' can be one of the most useful limits to apply. 'Clinical trial', 'meta-analysis' and 'randomized controlled trial' are all of importance to researchers and can be used to quickly identify key papers.

'Journal subsets' can sometimes be helpful if, for example, a search needs to be restricted to nursing journals only.

Box 13.3 Refining your search
- Make use of the wide range of limit commands to refine your search results
- Be careful not to over-limit, as you may miss relevant references
- Limiting to 'Abstracts' will omit editorials, which may be important

---

Combining sets

Many searches involve combining two or more MeSH headings, e.g. CORONARY DISEASE and EXERCISE. To do this you use three logical connectors AND, OR and NOT (also called Boolean operators).

- CORONARY DISEASE <u>AND</u> EXERCISE would retrieve papers indexed under both terms together.
- CORONARY DISEASE <u>OR</u> EXERCISE would give everything indexed under either term, individually. A useful mnemonic is 'OR gives you more'.

Although this sounds rather basic, it is easy to become confused during a long search involving many terms, and using the wrong operator can give some very strange results.

The third operator, NOT, can be useful in refining the results of a search. For example, you may be interested in papers on asthma in adults and not in children, so you could try this:

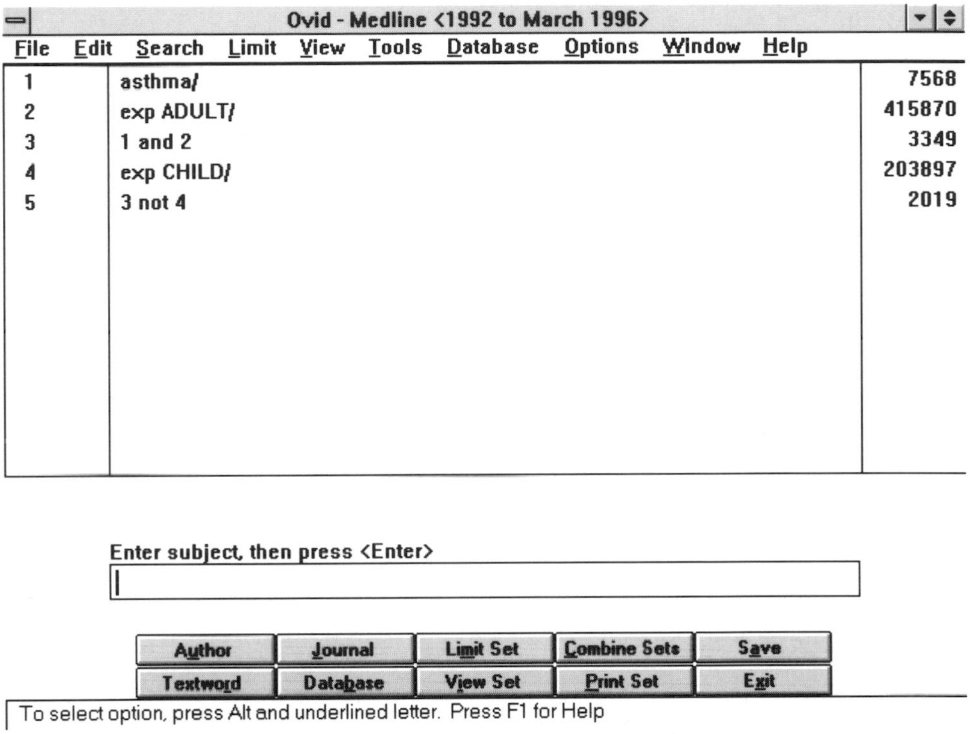

```
─|                        Ovid - Medline <1992 to March 1996>              |▼|⬍|
 File  Edit  Search  Limit  View  Tools  Database  Options  Window  Help
 1      asthma/                                                             7568
 2      exp ADULT/                                                        415870
 3      1 and 2                                                            3349
 4      exp CHILD/                                                       203897
 5      3 not 4                                                            2019
```

Enter subject, then press <Enter>

Author	Journal	Limit Set	Combine Sets	Save
Textword	Database	View Set	Print Set	Exit

To select option, press Alt and underlined letter. Press F1 for Help

Figure 13.4 Screenshot: Limiting sets.

The usual warning applies: **use with care lest you exclude too much**. This technique can help with cutting very large sets down to a manageable size. However, experiment with the operators AND, OR and NOT and note the different effects each has on your search results.

Searching individual fields

This option is accessed via the 'Search' menu on the top and bottom command lines and allows searching by 'Author' and 'Institution'.

Searching by 'Author'

Author searching prompts for the author's last name and first initial if known, and will retrieve all publications with that name. The truncation function can be used if you do not know the author's initials or full set of initials (this is also helpful, as a common problem is that an author may have papers published under several different forms of their name, with one, two, three or more initials) e.g. REYNOLDS, T$. Common names such as Smith or Jones inevitably cause problems, making author searching an inexact science in some cases.

Searching by 'Institution'

The institution is coded as the place of affiliation of the main author(s). This can be invaluable, particularly when the only definite thing you can remember about an important reference is that 'It was by some chap from Sheffield University'. Used in conjunction with subject, author or textword searching, a reference can often be retrieved from the scantiest of clues.

Saving search strategies

Once you have constructed a search strategy on a subject you may wish to use it again for updating references, or as the basis for a modified search. The strategy is the list of sets in numerical order. This can be saved to a floppy disk and used again (remember to name search files in a memorable manner).

Output from MEDLINE

There are two options once you have a set of references and have constructed your definitive set by marking chosen references:

- Print out all or selected references locally. This is useful if you do not require an electronic record, but have a lot of references. You are also less likely to lose the printout than scribbled notes on a scrap of paper.
- Download all or selected references to a floppy disk. There is usually a choice of downloading format offered. Downloading as a standard text file allows the list of references to be read into any wordprocessor. For personal bibliographic software choose the appropriate format and read it in.

BIDS allows users to send lists of references as text files via e-mail.

MANAGING REFERENCES

References can take on a life of their own and quickly become unmanageable. There is nothing more irritating than mislaying an important reference just when it is most needed. Therefore, be systematic from the start. Even so, this area is often a graveyard of good intentions.

The simplest method is 'paper only'. Keep lists of references in a legible form and file photocopies of what you feel are the major papers. Identifying a reference in a hurry will be a problem.

An advance on the above method is to use an indexing system – the most common is card file boxes. Each card might list the authors, title and journal, with a few handwritten notes on the paper. These can be indexed in a variety of ways, e.g. alphabetically by author or subject. As long as you understand the system, it should work. Most people also like to file copies of some of the papers.

Additionally, using a wordprocessing (WP) package you can store lists of references retrieved from a literature search so that you have legibility, some portability and easy 'cutting and pasting' into documents. However, the ways in which the data can be manipulated are restricted.

You could construct a reference database in a relational database package, but this is time-consuming and only for the diehard computer addict. Fortunately, commercial companies have gone to the trouble of doing this for you with personal bibliographic software packages.

Personal bibliographic software

Personal bibliographic software (PBS) is designed specifically to cater for the needs of researchers wishing to maintain large lists of references. They are specifically designed databases for reference storage and manipulation. Facilities usually available include:

- Manual entry of references
- Entry of references by downloading to disk from CD-ROM and online databases
- Adding comments to references
- Linking references to documents in a WP package using footnotes/endnotes
- Producing references in a variety of citation styles
- Retrieval and selection under many different search keys (e.g. author, date, subject)
- 'Look-up' lists of regularly used author and journal names.

Most PBS packages perform the above, although exact facilities will obviously vary between different packages.

The most readily available PBS packages are:

- Reference Manager (DOS, Windows and Macintosh)
- ProCite (DOS, Windows and Macintosh)
- EndNote (DOS, Windows and Macintosh)
- Papyrus (DOS; Macintosh version under development)

- Autobiblio (Macintosh)
- Refsys (DOS; Windows version under development).

The differences between the packages are far fewer than their similarities. The first three listed are all similarly priced (in the region of £250 excl. VAT). They all require an extra software add-on to enable downloading from different host systems ('capture software'). They also have an attractive interface and are relatively user-friendly.

Papyrus is currently only available in a DOS format and is consequently rather old-fashioned in appearance. It does, however, do everything the others do, and is able to import data without the need for add-on software. It has the advantage of being considerably cheaper than the others at £84 (excl. VAT). It is also approved by the Joint Academic Network (JANET) for general use in higher education environments. However, it is much more limited than the others when linked to WP documents. Autobiblio is Macintosh format only, but will capture downloaded references without additional software and costs £99 (incl. VAT). Refsys is produced by the same company for IBM PCs. It is less sophisticated than the Autobiblio and costs the same amount.

In spite of the intuitive way in which most of these packages operate, if you are used to using computer applications, it takes a while to learn all the facilities and to use them efficiently, but it is worth it.

As personal preference is so important with a piece of software that is likely to be in regular use, the best way to choose between the rival systems is to request a demonstration disk from the suppliers and give them a try. Remember to choose one which is compatible with your WP package.

Suppliers: (prices excl. VAT unless stated)

Reference Manager
Bilaney Consultants Ltd
St Julians
Sevenoaks
Kent
TN15 0RX

Tel: 01732 450002
Fax: 01732 450003

£250

(Capture software £100)

ProCite
PBS Europe
Woodside
Hinksey Hill
Oxford
OX1 5AU

Tel: 01865 326612
Fax: 01865 736354

£259

(Capture software £139. Bought together £299)

EndNote
Cherwell Scientific Publishing Ltd
The Magdalen Centre
Oxford Science Park
Oxford
OX4 4GA

Tel: 01865 784800
Fax: 01865 784801

£229

(Capture software £99. Bought
together £299)

Autobiblio and **Refsys**
Biosoft
22 Hills Road
Cambridge
CB2 1BJ

Tel: 01223 68622
Fax: 01223 312873

Both £99 incl. VAT

Papyrus
Software for Science Ltd
PO Box 28
Letchworth
Herts
SG6 2HP

Tel: 01462 488883
Fax: 01462 488886

£84

(includes capture software)

Further reading

Dickersin K, Scherer R and Lefebvre C (1994) Identifying relevant studies for systematic reviews. *BMJ*. **309**: 1286–91.

Jones RJ (1993) Personal computer software for handling references from CD-ROM and mainframe sources for scientific and medical reports. *BMJ*. **307**: 180–4.

Lee N *et al.* (1995) Storing and managing data on a computer. *BMJ*. **311**: 562–5.

Lindberg DA *et al.* (1993) Use of MEDLINE by physicians for clinical problem solving. *Journal of the American Medical Association*. **269**(24): 3124–9.

Lowe HJ and Barnett GO (1994) Understanding and using the medical subject headings (MeSH) vocabulary to perform literature searches. *Journal of the American Medical Association*. **271**(14): 1103–8.

Rowlands J *et al.* (1995) ABC of medical computing. Online searching. *BMJ*. **311**: 500–4.

Your local medical library should be able to offer you user's guides to MEDLINE and any other reference databases they subscribe to. Many medical libraries also offer training sessions.

14

The use of microcomputers in medical research

Michael Bannon

In this chapter I will attempt to provide a brief overview of the ways in which medical research might be enabled by the use of a computer. The approach given is a highly personalized one that I have developed over several years, and which seems to be appropriate to research I have been involved with. Throughout the chapter the term 'computer' refers to a microcomputer, i.e. one which is small enough to either sit on a desk or be carried around, but which is not necessarily small in processing power. The use of mainframe computers, which are large and usually situated in universities and other large organizations, will not be considered in any depth. It might be useful to first consider what a computer actually is and what it does.

WHAT IS A COMPUTER?

Computers have been defined as electronic digital devices which, under the control of a stored set of instructions (known as a program), automatically accept and process data and supply the results of that processing to a user. The physical components of a computer are known as its *hardware*, whereas the term *software* refers to the various programs in existence which enable computers to perform their processing tasks.

Hardware consists of:

- *Input devices*, such as keyboards, scanners or, rarely, voice input apparatus, which are used to submit data or instructions to the computer's processor. A mouse is also an input device, and is used to move the cursor or pointer on the computer screen
- A *central processing unit* (CPU), which acts as the 'nerve centre' of the computer and is where all computation takes place. The amount of data that can be handled by a computer and the speed at which they are processed together represent the power of the computer. Many technical terms are used to describe this power: first, the rate at which electronic pulses are sent from the processing is measured in MHz (megahertz: 1 MHz = 1 000 000 pulses/second), and secondly the size of the processor's memory (which is known as RAM, or random access memory), and this is measured in megabytes (Mb). The byte is the smallest storage unit used in computers
- *Storage devices* hold both data and programs until they are needed for processing. In addition, they also store the information produced after processing has taken place. A variety of storage media are in use, including magnetic tape and magnetic disks
- *Output devices* are responsible for transferring the results of processed data to the user, usually to a screen or via a printer.

The basic functions of any computer are as follows (Figure 14.1):

- Capture of data in a variety of formats from numerous sources
- Subsequent processing of data into useful information
- Storage of both data and information until they are required
- Production on demand of the results of both data and information processing.

A fundamental but important difference exists between the concepts of *data* and *information*. Data consist of facts, ideas or concepts which have not been organized

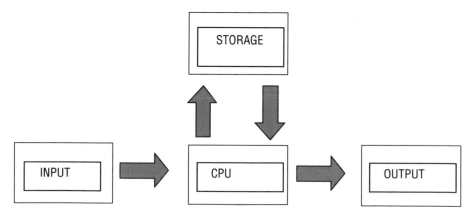

Figure 14.1 Basic components of a computer. Arrows refer to the flow of data.

or processed in any way, whereas information consists of data that have been processed in such a way that they become more meaningful for us.

The following example illustrates the inherent difference between the two concepts. Table 14.1 shows 51 intelligence quotients or gross quotients relating to a sample of children who attend a school for pupils with learning difficulties.

The numbers as they stand do not tell us much about the children concerned in terms of overall trend or averages. However, if these individual values were entered on to a statistical spreadsheet such as Minitab, then it would be quite feasible to perform simple calculations, as the following example shows. By simply typing the command 'describe GRO_QUO' we obtain the response shown in Figure 14.2.

We are made immediately aware that the GQ of the children studied ranges from 48 to 98 with a mean of 71.37, and that the median is close to the mean. In addition, we can graphically represent the spread of values around the mean by asking the computer to perform what is known as a dotplot, as shown in Figure 14.3.

Table 14.1 Gross quotients of 51 children with learning difficulties

60	66	80	87	66	67	76	77	83	79	75	59	59
83	75	71	65	81	84	50	72	65	68	70	72	60
86	58	77	86	48	78	68	59	48	76	91	98	67
65	82	76	52	88	74	72	65	84	65	66	61	

	Number	MEAN	MEDIAN	TRMEAN	STDEV	SEMEAN
Gro_quo*	51	71.37	72.00		71.49	11.36
1.59						

	MIN	MAX	Q1	Q3
Gro_quo	48.00	98.00	65.00	80.00

*Gro_quo = gross quotients

Figure 14.2 Statistical spreadsheet.

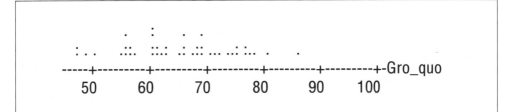

Figure 14.3 Dotplot.

Furthermore we can easily represent the data in the form of a histogram, as in Figure 14.4.

The computer and its software have converted the raw data into useful information for us. By performing other calculations upon these data we could easily learn more about the children being studied. It is possible to undertake such data analysis by manual means, but this becomes increasingly difficult when the number of subjects is large and the data become more complex.

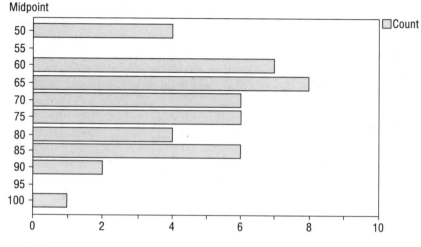

Figure 14.4 Histogram.

ADVANTAGES OF COMPUTERS IN RESEARCH

Computers have been used to some extent to successfully enhance aspects of clinical care, patient administration and computer-assisted learning. They can be similarly used to promote health care research, whether this is biomedical in orientation or is primary care or community in its focus. The use of a computer can bestow certain advantages to the researcher (Table 14.2).

Computers are capable of rapidly completing tasks which we would find difficult or even impossible. For example, many research projects involve the use of a questionnaire, which is administered to a target group of individuals. Good

Table 14.2 How computers can facilitate medical research

Accelerate and automate tasks which we would find difficult or even impossible to perform manually
Facilitate communication on a global scale
Time and project management
Reference management

questionnaire design is fraught with difficulty and a pilot study is usually undertaken first to ensure the appropriateness of the questions as well as their validity.

The overall aim of a project might be to determine patient satisfaction with outpatient services. It is not unusual to have access to the names, addresses and postcodes of several thousand patients which are stored on a computer. A pilot study could be undertaken by performing a mailshot to a 10% sample of the total target population. There are available to us numerous statistical tables which contain lists of random numbers, and hence we could randomly select 10% of the names and addresses by manual means. This might be an appropriate approach if the total target population were of the order of 100–200. A manual method becomes almost impossible if the total population to be surveyed is 1000–2000. Most databases and statistical packages contain a random function whereby it is possible to instruct the computer to select from the address list one record in ten. Furthermore, databases are able to produce the output of such an instruction in the form of an address label. We can then use a wordprocessing package to print the address labels and also a customized letter to accompany each questionnaire (Figure 14.5).

Communication between researchers is now achievable on a truly global scale via the Internet. It is now possible to communicate and exchange information with colleagues and institutions located on the other side of the world.

The completion of a successful research project requires (in addition to dedication, hard work and enthusiasm) considerable skills in time management. Some researchers already possess these skills in abundance. However, a significant

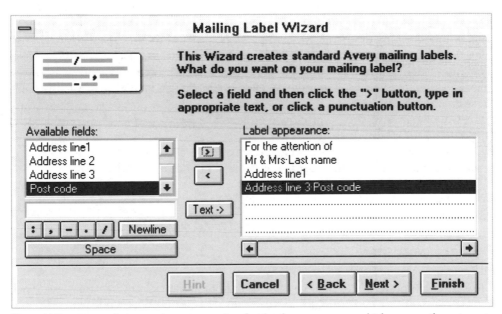

Figure 14.5 Microsoft Access is an example of a database program which can easily automate tasks such as the design of mailing labels from a database of names and addresses.

amount of medical research is undertaken by professionals who are not employed full time by an academic institution, and who strive to complete their project around the time constraints of full-time clinical work. This is difficult. During the course of any project of significant size or importance, an impressive list of useful and important contact names and addresses will develop. In addition, there will be significant deadlines to adhere to and important dates and appointments to keep in mind. There are a number of computerized personal organizers available which can greatly assist in time management. In addition, many computers come preloaded with personal information management software. Apart from effective management of one's own time, the overall project will need to be efficiently managed. There is an ethical obligation upon all researchers to do this, especially if funding has been provided for the project. A significant project is likely to be complex and to involve many different individuals, apart from the lead researcher. Indeed, most health care-related research is likely to be multidisciplinary in its approach. It is often necessary to employ one or more research assistants, to seek the advice of a statistician, or to collaborate in a significant manner with another academic department. This will ultimately add to the complexity of the project, and it is essential to maintain an overall oversight. Project management software is also available, which can be of great use. Apart from this, a Gantt chart can be easily constructed and continually updated by means of a wordprocessor.

A research project of any size will result in the accumulation of a large number of references. Most theses will contain several hundred references, consisting of published papers in professional journals, books, reports and other items. These will need to be efficiently indexed, stored and cross-referenced by theme. They should also be included in the main document in a standard format. This can be an onerous task when revisions are made to the text and the order of references needs to change as a result, or new references need to be added. Some of the latest wordprocessing packages, such as Word, are very helpful in this respect. Some universities also make use of software such as Reference Master or ProCite, which has been especially designed for this purpose.

It is worth making the point, however, that whether a manual or a computerized approach is adopted, a researcher must pay meticulous attention to detail.

So far we have discussed the main advantages of using a computer in a research project. It is now time to consider in some detail how they can be used.

Data input

Most research projects will involve the capture of data which will be stored and used later for analysis. The data might exist in the form of numbers, coded text, figures, diagrams or even photographic images. It is customary to develop some kind of proforma in order to record the data. The following is an example of a research project that required the recording of data which were available in a variety of formats.

The project aim was to study retrospectively the circumstances surrounding fatal childhood accidents over a ten-year period in a large district. To do this, it proved necessary to extract data from the local coroner's records. Although these contained considerable amounts of potentially useful data, stored in a fixed format, they were neither coded nor computerized. There was no alternative but to peruse the coroners' records manually and extract the relevant facts. In order to do this I designed a proforma (Figure 14.6). I then proceeded to copy the details of over 50 accidental deaths. Once this process was completed I began the laborious business of coding the data I had captured. Tedious calculations were also needed, which included exact determination of the ages of the children studied as well as distances from home to the place of the fatal accident. From the father's occupation I estimated socioeconomic groupings, and from the postcode I attempted to link the type of accident with known local indices of deprivation. From the data recorded under 'Accident details', I learnt more about the type of accident, the place of the accident and other important details. The resulting coded data were then entered in a numerical form on to a statistical package and then analysed. I became aware of the limitations of a manual approach:

- The data and information were not integrated
- Cross-referencing between individual records was difficult

Data Item	Format
Child s last name	Text
Child s first names	Text
Child s date of birth	Date
Child s address	Text
Postcode	Text
Date of accident	Date
Place of accident	Text
Time of accident	
Accident details	Text
Father s occupation	Text
Study number	Number

Figure 14.6 Proforma.

- The information became unwieldy when recorded on multiple sheets of paper, and several paper forms were lost and needed to be regenerated
- Manual tabulation of data was especially labour intensive.

I propose another approach, whereby the data are recorded electronically directly on to a personal computer using a database package. A database is a specialized type of software consisting of an integrated collection of records which can be interrogated and manipulated in a variety of ways. There are many commercial databases available at present, most of which are reasonably user-friendly. Within a database structure individual data items are entered in to fields, which together make up a record (Figure 14.7). A database file consists of a number of records, each of which must be uniquely identified. In the case of the accident study, data such as 'Child's last name', 'Date of birth' and so on represent discrete *fields*, which together make up a *record* relating to an individual child. A database *file* consists of the total number of records. A computer-generated proforma within a database is capable of accepting data in the form of numbers, characters, written text, and sometimes images. A database is capable of managing this task, as in Figure 14.8, where the form was created in Microsoft Access, a popular database package. The structure of the form is very like that of the manual paper form previously used for the same purpose.

The use of a database for the purpose of data entry and capture is strongly recommended for the following reasons:

- Databases can ensure that only valid data entries are accepted (i.e. we can specify that data entered lie within defined parameters)
- We can prevent duplicate records from being entered
- Coding of values can be facilitated
- Large numbers of records can be safely stored and retrieved when needed
- Most current database packages allow for the transcription of data into a variety of other software formats, such as statistical spreadsheets
- It is also possible to add new fields to the form at a later stage, and to create additional forms and link these to the original form
- Tedious manual calculation can be avoided (Access is capable of defining the age of each child at time of death by subtracting the fields 'Date of birth' from 'Date of accident' and providing the answer in days, months or years; in addition, it would have been feasible to export the postcodes of each child's address as well as the place of accident to a geographical information system, where distances could be accurately and quickly calculated).

Data field	⇒			
Data field	⇒	Record	⇒	Database file
Data field	⇒			

Figure 14.7 Database structure.

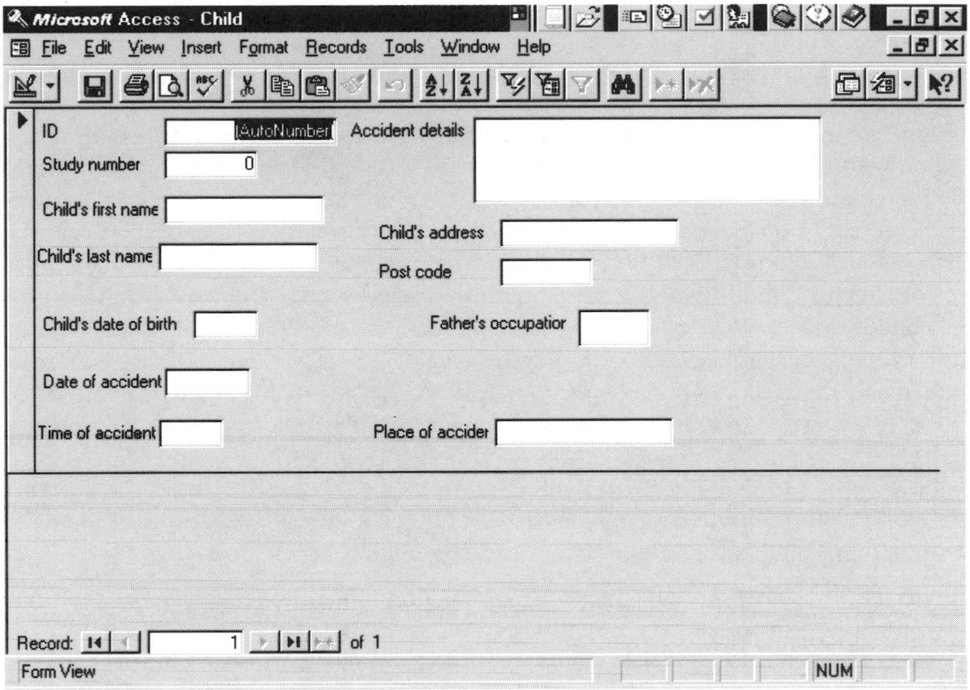

Figure 14.8 Form created in Microsoft Access for the purpose of data entry.

DATA ANALYSIS

Once data are captured they will require analysis. This can be undertaken quantitatively or qualitatively.

Quantitative analysis

This is concerned with data that are essentially in the form of measurements which can be subjected to statistical analysis. The intelligence quotients demonstrated earlier would represent an example of quantitative data. In general, statistical packages are used to analyse the results of quantitative research. There are several well respected statistical packages available which are eminently suitable for use on a PC, and the facilities provided include:

- Exploratory data analysis
- Summarizing data
- Analysis of variance
- Correlation and regression
- Survival analysis

- Calculation of sample size and power.

SPSS is a comprehensive package which is capable of providing a wide range of analyses and there are versions available for PCs that operate within the Windows environment. Minitab is also popular, and allows the user the choice of either pull-down menus or simple commands which can be typed. Many academic institutions will have arrangements whereby bona-fide students may purchase versions of these packages at reduced rates. EPI-INFO is also worthy of consideration. It has the advantage of being in the public domain, which means that users may make copies of the software and distribute it widely free of charge. EPI-INFO version 6 is now available, and consists of an integrated package of wordprocessor, database and numerous statistical tools. It is important to take full advantage of these packages and make them work for you. Most statistical software will possess the ability to perform *macros*, i.e. will automate the steps needed in the execution of common tasks. Most will also record the results of a session as an ASCII text file, which can be later incorporated into a document created with a wordprocessor. The analysis undertaken using Minitab at the beginning of this document was stored as a text file and then imported into the main document.

Analysis of qualitative data

This concerns not the examination of numerical data but rather the production of accurate descriptions based on face-to-face knowledge of individuals or social groups. On this occasion data collection is involved in objective reporting of opinions, views and personal feelings. Open-ended questions are often used in structured interviews, focus group discussions or self-completed questionnaires. This will generate large volumes of text. A number of qualitative analytical methods are available which include content analysis and the definition of themes. More recently software packages have been developed for the analysis of language, and these can facilitate this process. Such software is not yet widely available for PCs, but text can be appropriately exported to such packages by means of a wordprocessor.

DATA STORAGE

Computers are really useful for storing impressive amounts of data and information. A variety of storage media are available, including the computer's hard disk, floppy disks and tapes. However, careful consideration must be given to the security of the information stored on an individual computer, and this is particularly relevant when the information relates to patients. Many researchers prefer to use a portable computer such as a notebook or laptop. Despite offering considerable convenience, however, such machines are easily stolen and one must have a contingency plan for such disasters. Passwords can be incorporated into most software applications.

It is essential that data are stored in a neat and logical fashion in appropriate directories and subdirectories. A research project of any size will involve data and information that need to be stored together, rather like documents in individual folders which are then located in filing cabinets (Figure 14.9). For example, we could have one major directory named 'Research', with relevant subdirectories for literature searches, protocol and so on. There is no absolute way in which directories and subdirectories should be organized: the important principle is that a structure does exist, so that relevant files can be easily found and retrieved.

I also recommend that time be spent at regular intervals on various housekeeping chores, which may seem tedious but in the long term they will prove to be essential. The first task involves keeping the directories and their contents tidy. It will prove necessary from time to time to delete obsolete files, rename other files and to create new subdirectories. Secondly, backing up of data should be a regular routine. Imagine how you would cope if your computer or your files were no longer available as a result of theft, breakdown or accidental erasure. Backup of files can be easily achieved by means of floppy disks. If you can afford it, and if your project involves a large amount of data, then a tape storage device could prove to be invaluable.

I also advise that you make a system disk for your computer and keep it safe. A system disk contains vital files (including autoexec.bat and config.sys) which are needed to boot-up or start your computer. Sometimes these files can be altered accidentally or become corrupted, in which case your computer will not be able to start whichever operating system it uses.

Finally, one should be constantly vigilant for the possibility that the computer could become infected with a computer virus. Viruses are illegal, self-replicating computer programs which have been maliciously written to damage software, stored information or even the hard disk. Install an antivirus kit on your hard disk and meticulously check any floppy disk before copying it; this routine should also be extended to new software. If your computer is connected to a network you need to be especially careful.

PRODUCTION OF INFORMATION

At some stage in a project a progress report may be needed; an abstract may need submission to an academic meeting, and the final results will be written as a paper or a thesis. Wordprocessors were among the earliest software to be used

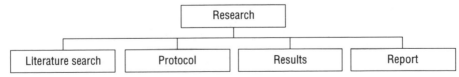

Figure 14.9 Directories and subdirectories.

on PCs. Current wordprocessors such as Word for Windows, WordPerfect and Ami-Pro possess advanced authoring features which include page numbering, chapter formation and reference management.

Desktop publishing software such as Harvard Graphics, Freelance Graphics or PowerPoint can produce graphs, graphics and illustrations, which greatly enhance the appearance of a thesis. They are also necessary for the creation of quality overheads and slides. The standard of presentation of theses has, in my experience, improved dramatically over recent years as a result of these tools.

What is needed for a research project

Components of the following will be needed:

- Wordprocessor
- Desktop publisher
- Database
- Statistical package
- Personal organizer.

Some integrated packages (e.g. Microsoft Office, Lotus Smartsuite) are available containing most of the above, and are often preloaded on newly purchased computers.

What computers cannot do

Although computers are powerful information processing devices they should be considered as tools to facilitate research, rather than as electronic oracles. They cannot turn a flawed research idea into a good one, nor can they rescue invalid data. In particular, they are unable to interpret data and the results of analysis in a truly meaningful way: this is still the responsibility of the human expert. It has been said that medicine is both an art and a science, requiring both intuitive skills and scientific knowledge. The same principle applies to medical research. As one writer has commented: 'The real danger of the computer age is not that computers will think like people but that people will think like computers' (Frank Romero).

Box 14.1 Tips for success
- Make regular backups of your files
- Maintain a neat set-up of directories and subdirectories
- Make a system disk for your computer
- Install a virus-checker and check all floppy disks before copying files from them

Further reading

Brown RA and Beck JS (1994) *Medical Statistics on Personal Computers*. BMJ Publishing Group, London.

Lowe D (1993) *Planning for Medical Research*. Astraglobe, Cardiff.

Norris DE, Skilbeck M, Hayward AE and Torpy DM (1985) *Microcomputers in Clinical Practice*. John Wiley, Chichester.

Polgar S and Thomas SA (1988) *Introduction to Research in the Health Sciences*. Churchill Livingstone, Melbourne.

Software

SPSS can be obtained from
SPSS UK Ltd
SPSS House
London Street
Chertsey
KT16 8AP

Minitab is available from
CleCom
Research Park
97 Vincent Drive
Birmingham B15 2SQ

EPI-INFO is usually available from most universities

15

Online research

Martin Wilkinson

One of the problems of research for general practitioners is their relative isolation from like-minded individuals and academic bodies. Often spare time is spent catching up with journals, and holidays are sacrificed to complete literature searches in distant medical libraries. Few are lucky enough, or have the resources, to have a comprehensive practice library. With the advent of the Internet, however, we have the world's literature at our fingertips. Complete literature searches can be carried out, references downloaded and printed, all from one's surgery. Regular dialogue is possible with others with similar academic interests both here and abroad, without leaving home. It is now possible, with practice, to find information about anything (well almost) during your surgery coffee break.

The aim of this chapter is:

- To introduce the Internet
- To explain how to go online
- To illustrate some of the applications for primary care research
- To warn the reader against possible pitfalls.

HISTORY OF THE INTERNET

There is no official history of the Internet, but 'Netties' speak of roots in 1960s military intelligence research. The US Defense Department had a computer network called the ARPAnet and wished to link radio and satellite computers in order to exchange intelligence. The first network was between four sites in 1969. Immediately the problem of computer compatibility prevented widespread development. Different computer systems were unable to understand each other, so with the ARPAnet came the first Internet protocol (IP). Each computer signal was translated into this common protocol before being transmitted.

> **Box 15.1 Online research**
> FG is a male patient of mine, aged 66, who has been slowly developing motor weakness of his left hand over the past six months. The weakness has been progressive and there is now suspicion of a similar weakness developing in his right arm and both legs. After seeking a neurological opinion Mr G came to see me for an explanation of the diagnosis given by the specialist: 'multifocal motor neuropathy'. To be honest, I had never heard of this and had difficulty explaining what it was. I explained my dilemma and suggested that a quick look in the practice library would solve the problem. I was surprised, and a little reassured, that my area of ignorance was not listed in *The Oxford Textbook of Medicine*. Unperturbed, I explained that I would find some information and contact Mr G later.
>
> After surgery I dialled into the MEDLINE database using my portable computer and modem. I searched the world literature back to 1966 and found just 16 references to multifocal motor neuropathy. Within ten minutes of dialling in I had the abstracts downloaded on to my hard disk. Using a wordprocessor I then collated the articles, deleted unwanted text and translated them into plain English to produce a summary of the world literature in the form of a patient information leaflet. I posted it to Mr G the next day. His neurologist found this information most useful at the next outpatient appointment.

In 1973 the network became international (*inte*rnational *net*work), with links to Norway and the UK. Academic institutions began to connect to ARPAnet, but international proliferation was limited by lack of international agreement on a protocol until 1982. During this time many commercial organizations had developed their own extensive networks, e.g. Hoover. These separate networks were linked into a new network, the National Science Foundation (NSFNET), an agency of the US government, and allowed communication to all other computers on the network and access to supercomputers and national databases. The NSF expanded access from computer boffins and military intelligence to universities and schools.

Today most academic institutions within the developed world have Internet access, and the commercial Internet service providers are encouraging private and business use. Worldwide there are now over 20 million users with direct access, 30 million e-mail addresses, 8 million university connections and 6 million commercial users. The size is doubling every few months, encouraged by ever-cheaper technology and commercial potential.

HOW DOES IT WORK?

The Internet is composed of millions of computers worldwide connected together by land lines, telephone cables, radio and satellite links. The computer signal is dissected into millions of data packets and these are directed from one computer to another using the IP as an address label. Data packets (like parcels in the post) are passed on to a sorting computer, which reroutes the 'mail' to the next best computer, and so on until the data packet reaches its receiver. My e-mail address is WILKIMJB@bham.ac.uk. A data packet sent to me from Australia will, for example, go to UK sorting office (UK), the universities network (ac), then to Birmingham University (bham), then to me (WILKIMJB). The route taken may vary, depending on which parts of the network are overloaded or fully operational.

The Internet has many features and possibilities, and I will describe those most likely to be used by the medical researcher, including:

- e-mail
- Telnet
- FTP
- Databases
- User groups
- The World Wide Web.

I have tried to give a taste of the Internet, with some suggestions for launching yourself into medical cyberspace. For those who seek more detail I recommend that they turn to Krol (1994).

GETTING ONLINE

To get on to the Internet you will require a personal computer (PC), a modem, a telephone socket and an account with an Internet service provider. Any modern PC can be used, although some of the more advanced features of the commercial services will only be available to those with the equivalent of an Intel 386, 4 Mb RAM and Window/Windows 95 or any colour Apple Mac with 8 Mb RAM . The more advanced features include sound, high-resolution graphics and video, and for these an Intel 486 or Pentium PC with 8 Mb (Windows) or 16 Mb (Windows 95) will be required. Most high street electrical retailers sell computers that more than satisfy these requirements, including a modem and software, for a price of around £1000.

For those outside universities plugging into the Internet will be via a telephone socket. A modem is needed to translate the computer signal to a telephone signal, and plugs between the computer and the socket. Modems have different speeds, from 1200 baud to 56 000 baud. This is important because a file may take 30 seconds to transfer at the faster rate but several frustrating minutes at the slowest rate, with a consequently larger phone bill. The ultimate speed is also limited by the Internet service provider, but it is not uncommon to have 28 000 baud access and this should be the minimum standard when buying a new modem.

SOFTWARE

Academic departments have free access via their departmental computer network, linked to the university system. Academics (lecturers and students) are also entitled to an e-mail address. The rest of us have to subscribe to a commercial online service. The information management and technology strategy of the NHS is bringing forth the possibility of e-mail addresses for all GP practices, and this will include a gateway to the Internet via the NHS network.

Internet software is often offered free with new modems, allowing easy installation and free access on a trial basis to one of the commercial online services. All services cost money, for both telephone time and access time. As a rule, the bigger commercial services are easier to use, have more advanced features and allow full Internet access. The larger providers have local access with local call charges. The cheaper, more limited sites have the full Internet features but are not so user-friendly, have an unattractive screen appearance, and may be limited to long-distance telephone charges. Unfortunately, many rely on you giving credit card details and they take money from your credit card account directly, depending on your monthly use. Security is by password, so it is in your and your bank balance's interest not to let anyone use your password.

The full software package and updates can usually be downloaded via your modem from the Internet, or sent on floppy disk. Several providers are listed below. The market is very competitive, so it would be wise to check prices and features before having a free trial – after giving your credit card details it may not be so simple to cancel. One of the many Internet magazines will have details of all the current providers for comparison. The ideal Internet service provider would have:

- Many existing subscribers (for its own user groups, continued development and features)
- Full Internet access (Telnet, FTP, WWW, Usenet)
- Your own Web page space
- 28 800 bps access or ISDN (integrated services digital network)
- Local access
- Easy-to-use software
- e-mail
- Low charges, suited to your potential use.

e-MAIL

e-mail is probably the most common use for the busy primary care researcher, and in its simplest form is a very easy and efficient way of sending a letter to another computer (Figure 15.1). The addressee can either read the message off their

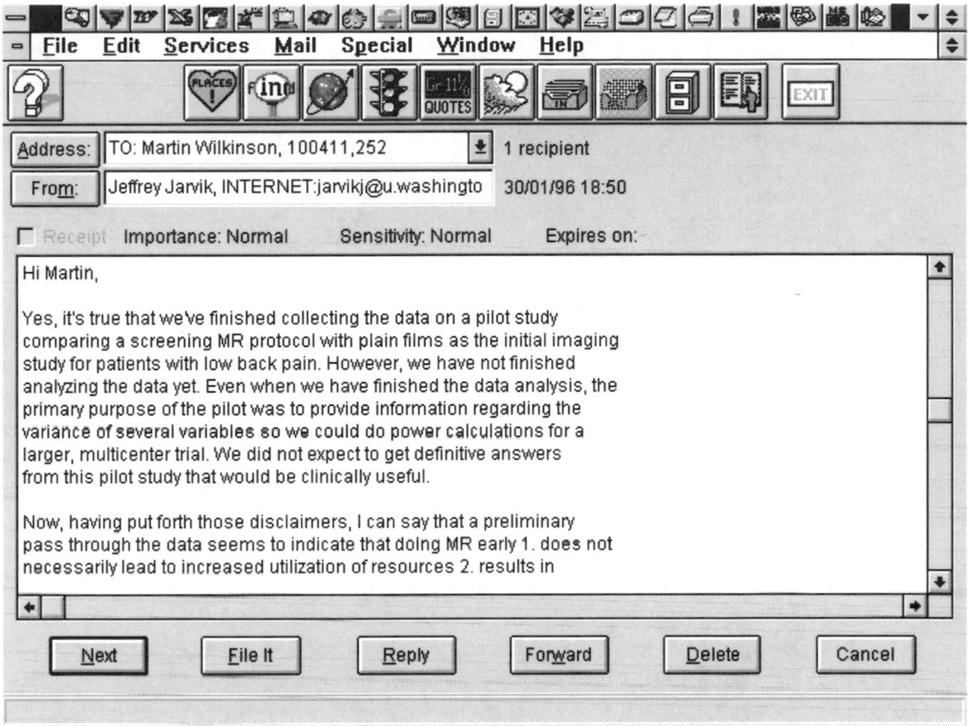

Figure 15.1 An e-mail message sent by the CompuServe Information Manager.

computer screen or print it on to paper. e-mail is much faster than the postal system but is slower than a fax, taking anything from a few seconds to several hours to arrive. The electronic post cannot be read, and the addressee is unaware of its presence until they go online and look in their electronic mailbox. If they rarely do this then a fax or traditional letter would be better.

An electronic letter allows the message to be imported and manipulated in a wordprocessor, and can be posted on with seamless corrections or additions. Copies can be sent at the click of a mouse button to individuals or, for example, to members of your local research club. Faxes are quicker if seconds count, and usually the communications software included in your system will allow the sending of faxes as well as e-mail. A separate fax machine is therefore unnecessary.

Files can be attached to e-mail letters and be sent with them, for example spreadsheet data, wordprocessor data or complete computer programs. e-mail between different Internet service providers may cause the attached file to be scrambled, as they could use different protocols to transmit the letter. To overcome this problem a facility should be offered to translate the file into a universal format (encoding) before transmission, unless the addressee uses the same Internet provider and hence protocol. One well recognized format is ASCII, which is a simple text file understood by most computers. The exchange of whole computer programs is easier between the same Internet service provider or by using a bulletin board service (see below).

e-mail is not confidential, possibly being read en route by various system administrators. People also have a habit of saving e-mail letters, unintentionally, and often for years, with regular duplicated backups. Your letter may turn up in years to come, so be polite and do not commit anything to e-mail that you do not wish to be made public.

TELNET

Telnet is an application that allows you to execute commands on a remote computer as if you were logged on locally. In order to make a successful Telnet connection you need to know the name of the computer site and have a valid user name and password for that site. Once logged on you can use the remote computer to access databases or local networks. The level of access is usually governed by a password. It is possible to use the remote computer to log on to other remote computers, and this is how computer hackers avoid detection, by using a distant computer to do their hacking. The legal use is to remotely log on to public services, library indexes and databases. Interestingly, if your Internet service provider is not recognized as a valid user of one remote system, you may well be able to 'log in' from another public access computer that is recognized (e.g. JANET).

There are many worldwide public access computers that allow remote log in. Possibly the most useful as a GP researcher is the BMA library computer at BMA headquarters. This computer has a full MEDLINE database back to 1966. Full MEDLINE utilities are available and the search result can be saved to your hard disk. To gain access one has to log into, or 'Telnet' to JANET, the Joint Academic Network of educational establishments in the UK. For example using a Windows-based Internet service provider, all the user has to do is point the mouse and click on the Telnet box and, when instructed, enter 'X25-pad.ja.net'. The remote computer asks for you to log in and you enter 'Janet', then you need a password: again, 'Janet' gains entry. From this remote computer you will be asked where you want to connect to and you enter 'uk.org.bma' and use the password 'VT100'; you are then logged into the computer at the BMA library ready to use MEDLINE. Unfortunately, you will then need a further login name and password, which are available only to BMA members. Another way in is to connect via Telnet, first to 'sun.nsf.ac.uk' then 'uk.bma.org'. All this is quite slow, and if you are a regular user it is quicker to dial direct into the BMA computer using a standard communications package such as Norton PC-anywhere. The Internet route is slower, but at local call rates; the direct route is a London telephone call but a faster rate of data transfer.

For further information about the BMA MEDLINE service, software requirements and a password, contact Jane Rowlands at the BMA Library, Tel 0171 383 6224.

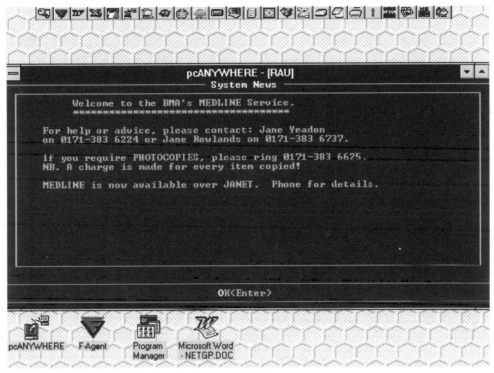

Figure 15.2 Remote access of MEDLINE via BMA library.

Box 15.2 Archie

I would like to contact other general practitioners in the UK interested in rheumatology for a research project. Using CompuServe, a Windows-based, commercial network, I click the 'Professional' icon designating professional usergroups, which in turn leads me to 'UK-Professional' forum. I enter the private 'doctors' lounge', where only bone fide medics are allowed. Here I find several of my colleagues who I invite to a conference (Figure 15.3). They appear on my screen and we begin a live conference swapping information and ideas. I am in the comfort of my study and they are dotted about the UK and the world. Finally, using FTP without knowing it, I upload my rheumatology questionnaire to the library for others to use. While in the library I see a coronary risk score programme and download to use when undertaking new patient screening.

FILE TRANSFER AND USERGROUPS

Usergroups and bulletin board services (BBS) allow special interest groups to hold meetings, leave messages and access specialist libraries. Usergroups are on the

Internet, whereas bulletin board services are accessed via a direct telephone number to the bulletin board computer concerned and are not linked to the Internet. There are over 13 000 usergroups on the Internet, limited only by your imagination.

File transfer protocol (FTP) is a common protocol allowing file transfer from one computer to another. There are many areas on the Internet where interested groups keep computer programs, graphics and documents for others to download to their own computer. FTP is easier with the Windows-based Internet Service providers who often have their own file-searching tools (file finders) and usergroups. On the Internet a popular file finder is Archie, found by 'Telnet-ing' to an Archie server (archie.doc.ic.ac.uk, Login: Archie) – however, this is for the more experienced user. File finders search for programs by file type, e.g. graphics files or GIF files, or by key word.

SYSTEM:	Kate Thomas has entered the group
Joyce Kenkre:	Hello, Kate, Congrats on the MD. Would you be interested in the rheumatology survey?
Roger Holder:	Your figures are totally meaningless, sorry!
Yvonne Carter:	Hello Kate. I was thinking we could involve more practices
Joyce Kenkre:	Don't worry, Roger, I think my computer scrambled the results.
System:	Martin Wilkinson has left the group
Kate Thomas:	Yes, I will discuss it at the practice meeting, how many practices do you need?

Figure 15.3 A live conference in the UK-Professional forum.

THE WORLD WIDE WEB

The World Wide Web (WWW) is the most exciting development of the Internet and has largely superseded other Internet navigation tools and information services such as Gopher and WAIS. It was originally developed by CERN, the European Particle Physics Laboratory. The Web is based on a technology called 'hypertext' which allows selected words in a text to link to other documents and provides a very easy means of navigating the Internet. The Web exists in the form of pages, 'Web pages', which usually include pictures and text. Often the pictures themselves are 'hypermedia', i.e. similar to hypertext, so clicking on different parts of a picture directs the user to associated documents or Web pages. Information can be left and files or graphics downloaded. Many original FTP and Telnet sites now have their version of WWW pages which are much simpler to use.

In the medical world there are a multitude of Web pages, but only a few are worth accessing. Anyone can set-up a Web page and consequently there is a lot of junk out there which can take many frustrating minutes to sift through. Various search 'engines' are available, e.g. Lycos, which allow key word searches often revealing hundreds of possible Web sites. Fortunately there are many high quality medical index Web pages which guide the user to the quality pages.

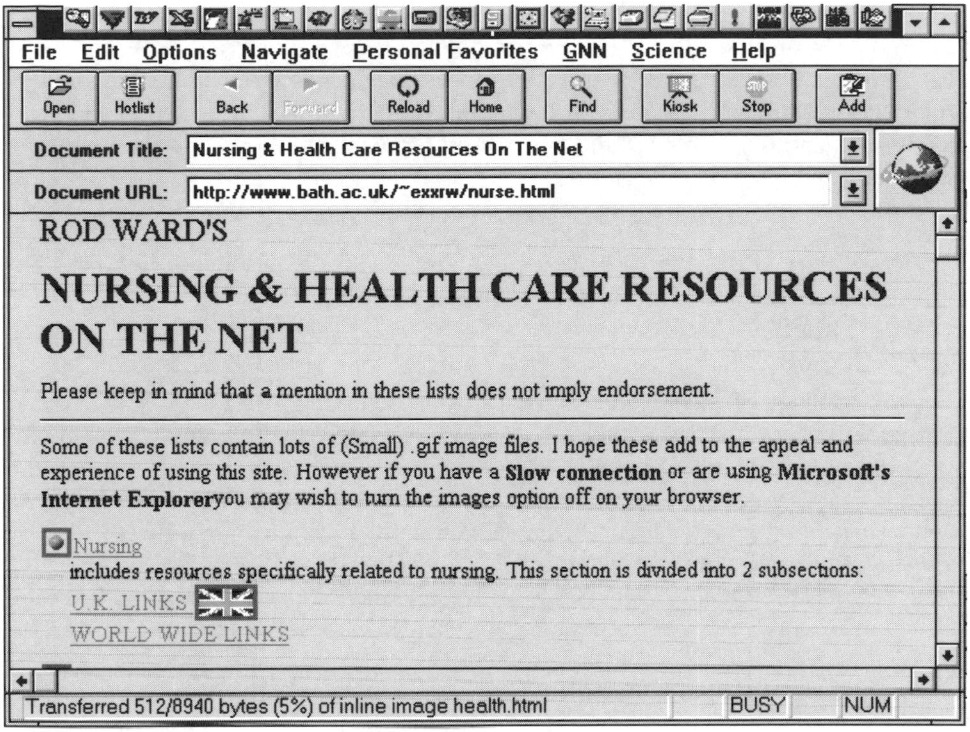

Figure 15.4 Nursing & Health Care Resources Web page.

Web pages now exist for several journals including the *British Medical Journal* and the *Nursing Standard*. These allow access to previous articles which often can be downloaded to disk either in full or abstract form. Many journal sites invite contributions and letters via Web page e-mail links. The use of the page being simplicity itself but often very slow.

Many academic units have their own Web sites with details of staff, courses and downloadable files. Hospitals, research networks and special interest groups have recently come online. The Cochrane Collaboration Web page is a fast growing site with a multitude of information about evidence-based medicine and the latest reviews. Other interesting sites include a virtual hospital in Iowa and serial MRI scans at Harvard University which allows a virtual trip through the body in time and space.

A HEALTH WARNING – VIRUSES

A computer virus is a relatively small program that gets on to the hard disk without invitation or announcement. It lies in wait and declares itself when least suspected often with disastrous results – wiping your hard disk for example. Most viruses are self-replicating and are getting increasingly difficult to detect. According to the USA National Computer Security Association, 65% of viruses are passed on from floppy disks, 25% from local networks and 7% from Internet usage. It is imperative that you protect yourself from viruses if you intend to access the Internet. The consequences may be damage not only to your own computer but the surgery computer network as well.

Simple precautions will make infections less likely:

- Do not leave floppy disks in the drive on turning off the computer or re-booting.
- Be selective about who uses your computer, use passwords.
- Install antiviral software.
- Make regular back-ups.

Antiviral software should be used to scan the computer on a regular basis and all new and foreign disks scanned before use, ideally on a 'quarantine' computer isolated from the surgery network. Most scanners now run continuously in the background to detect virus-like activity. As some new viruses target the scanners themselves the software needs regular updates, for example quarterly, to identify new strains. The best virus scanners available include Dr Solomon, Norton Antivirus and F-Protect. F-protect is available as shareware and can be downloaded from the net with bi-monthly updates, using a file finder search for fprot.exe.

Further information and useful Internet sites (UK telephone numbers)

Internet Service Providers:

America On-line	0800 279 1234
CompuServe	0800 289378
Demon Internet	0181 371 1234
Europe On-line	0171 331 4692
eWorld	0800 868206
Microsoft Network	0345 002000
Planet Internet	0500 345400
Pipex Dial	0500 474739
UK OnLine	01749 333300

Recommended Web pages

Archives of Family Medicine Homepage	http://www.ama-assn.org/journals/standing/fami/famihome.htm
The Electronic Journal of Informatics in Primary Care	http://www.ncl.ac.uk/~nphcare/PHCSG/Journal/sept95/sept1.htm
Bandolier	http://www.jr2.ox.ac.uk:80/Bandolier/

BMJ	http://www.bmj.com/bmj/
Centre For Medical Education: :Web update	http://www.dundee.ac.uk/meded/webupdate/
Cochrane Collaboration	http://hiru.mcmaster.ca:80/cochrane/ cochrane.htm
Description of Clinical Practice Guideline Abstracts	http://hiru.mcmaster.ca/cpg/abstract.htm
Family practice	http://www.uib.no/isf/guide/family.htm
General EBM Resources	http://cebm.jr2.ox.ac.uk/docs/otherebmgen .html
GP-UK Home Page	http://www.ncl.ac.uk/~nphcare/GPUK/ gpuktemp.html
Health Information Research Unit	http://hiru.mcmaster.ca/
Essential Resources	http://www.ama-assn.org/med_link/peer.htm
JAMA	http://www.ama-assn.org/journals/standing/ jama/jamahome.htm
Lycos Search 'engine'	http://www.lycos.com/
National Library of Medicine	http://www.nlm.nih.gov/
Nurse	http://medsrv2.bham.ac.uk/nursing/
Nursing & Health Care Resources	http://www.bath.ac.uk/~exxrw/nurse.html
Nursing Standard On-line	http://www.csv.warwick.ac.uk:8000/ejournal/
University of Birmingham, UK	http://www.bham.ac.uk:80/
Yahoo directory of WWW	http://www.yahoo.com/

Further reading

Krol E (1994) *The Whole Internet – Users' Guide and Catalogue* (2nd edn.) O'Reilly & Associates Inc., Sebastopal, California.

16

Getting published

John Skelton

Many people undertake research because they believe they have something interesting to say, many others because it helps their career; most researchers are driven by both these motives. Either way, research is meaningless without publication, and getting published is something that requires thought.

Standards of academic writing vary enormously. Some people write very well naturally. Some are very weak – in a very few cases to the point where their writing can make them appear confused or stupid. This chapter invites you to look at what is involved in writing up a study for publication. It says nothing about the content of what you write. It assumes that you have completed a study and want to know how to present it to a journal editor in a form that will carry conviction.

There are three ways in which a consideration of the writing process might benefit an individual. For weak writers it can show them 'how to'. They can be given models, hints, bits and pieces of practical advice. To a limited extent they can be given a template. Strong writers are unlikely to benefit in this very direct way, but they can be rendered more aware, more conscious of the successful strategies they pursue. This ability to articulate will in turn enable them to introspect, and to evaluate their own work and that of others. Finally, an awareness of how academic writing is put together can help you to read the work of others more easily.

CONVENTIONS IN READING AND WRITING

A lot of what has been written about academic writing is, unfortunately, vacuous exhortation (be simple! be clear!) with no description of what these things are – simplicity is, inevitably, a complex concept in any case. This chapter therefore has an entirely different starting point, one which is commonplace in the teaching of reading and writing, but I think more or less unknown in medicine: the fact that successful writing for publication is a matter of getting a good study and then learning the rules of the academic writing game. The key point is that medical journal writing is a very highly conventionalized genre.

The most famous of all descriptions of reading is that it is 'a psycholinguistic guessing game' (Goodman and Fleming 1969). In other words, good readers make guesses as they go along about what is likely to come next. You might like to see how this works by playing what is known as 'Kim's game'. Cover up completely the text in Box 16.1, then reveal it to yourself a word at a time, trying as you do so to guess what word will come next. The text is the opening of an extremely well-known fairy story – and as you guess the last word you'll see which one.

You will see that your guesses are directed by your expectations – of what the world is like, of what the conventions of fairy stories are. Your guesses, then, are informed by *schema* (originally in Bartlett 1932, but much used in reading/writing theory since the 1960s).

Incidentally, if you fail to understand a text it is very probably not principally a matter of unfamiliar technical terms, but of relevant schema: you come to the text without particular expectations and have no context to fit it into. This accounts for the phenomenon you may well have noticed: that you read a text in an unfamiliar subject, understand more or less every word, but still have the feeling that it does not make sense.

What can we conclude from this? If you are writing in a particular genre you are under contract to follow particular conventions. If you do not, your work may seem naive or incomprehensible. Except that:

- *Adequate* writing is a matter of modest obedience
- *Good* writing *may* involve sensitive breaches of convention.

Rules are for the obedience of the weak and the guidance of the strong.

CONVENTIONS IN MEDICAL WRITING

In what follows I shall look at the conventions that are typical of relatively highbrow medical writing. Some conventions are made explicit by the International Committee of Medical Journal Editors, and you should be aware of these. Others are a matter of house style, vary from journal to journal, and are printed in some or all issues of the journal under the heading 'Notes to contributors', or a similar title. What I am concerned with, however, are conventions which are not so explicit.

There are certain conventions that everyone quietly acknowledges but which are seldom discussed. In particular:

- Almost all contemporary scientific writing is ostensibly factual and depersonalized
- Almost all contemporary scientific writing ostensibly recounts experiments which went fairly smoothly.

Box 16.1 Kim's game

Once

upon

a

time

there

lived

in

a

certain

city

of

China

an

impoverished

tailor

who

had

a

son

called

Aladdin

In fact, of course, scientific writing takes place in an often highly competitive environment, with research money and people's jobs at stake; it is undertaken by fallible people with occasional axes to grind. It is not exactly improbable that there is a discrepancy between what is written (a regal progress to victory) and what actually happened. Gilbert and Mulkay (1984) are very good on the way in which a polished academic phrase ('A random sample of participants was selected') can conceal a dingier reality ('We were dragging people off the street by the end of it all').

To labour the obvious, perhaps, this sort of thing deserves to be construed as humour rather than cynicism. More seriously, there is a quite straightforward sense in which scientific articles in general do not tell the whole truth. To take a very obvious example, it is very rare indeed for an experiment to be replicable purely as a result of reading an article. Journal space does not usually permit the luxury of, for example, publication of all the results obtained, or all the questions asked in a questionnaire. In other words, when you write it is not your purpose to tell the whole truth (an impossible task) but to imply your credibility. You do this by showing that you know the rules, i.e. the conventions, by which the game is played.

MOVE STRUCTURE

An analysis of move structure is an analysis of the kind of things that are likely to occur in particular circumstances (for details of the methodology, see Swales 1990 and Skelton 1994). An analysis of doctor–patient consultations might well conclude that the following moves, among others, were very likely to happen:

- Greeting/farewell
- Description by patient of problem
- Evaluation by doctor of patient problem
- Doctor statement on management of problem.

Relatively unlikely to occur might be:

- Accusation by patient of professional incompetence

and so on.

The remainder of this chapter is concerned with an analysis of the typical move structure of work accepted in the 'Original papers' section of such journals as the *British Medical Journal* and the *British Journal of General Practice*. Let me stress that a move structure analysis of a genre will come up with what *tends* to happen, not what always happens, and certainly not what *must* happen. You would have to resign yourself to a fairly long search before you found an article which was an exact fit with what is described below.

The examples I have used to exemplify introductions are brief, minimal statements of what is required. To exemplify the other sections I have chosen just two papers, for ease of reference, both somewhat discursive, to show how this minimal picture may be fleshed out by the authors' requirements.

The best-researched and understood part of the research article is the Introduction (you may be surprised to learn that it has been analysed to the point of exhaustion: see especially Swales 1990, although what follows is an adaptation of an earlier version of work recounted there). It is argued that many research articles in all disciplines, but particularly in the sciences, have Introduction sections which aim to 'create a research space' (Swales 1990) and do four things. First, they *assert that the study is **important**, or **central**, perhaps because the problem to be discussed is **frequent**.* Secondly, they *discuss previous research.* Thirdly, they *indicate a gap in the research with a word/phrase like **however**, **little is known*** or by *identifying a question with a word like **suggest***, and finally they *make a promise to **describe** what was **undertaken**,* or they *state the **aim** or **purpose** of the study.* Box 16.2 gives two examples.

The structure of the Introduction and the Discussion sections of academic articles is to a considerable degree governed by stylistic convention. The structure of the Method and Results sections is more variable, because it is driven almost entirely by the experimental design which the former section describes. Nevertheless, there are general patterns. The function of the Method section, for instance, is to *describe the procedures used and assert their credibility,* whereas the function of the Results section is *to describe (but not discuss) relevant figures in an apparently transparent and objective manner.* Some of the conventions here are given in Box 16.3.

Finally, there is the Discussion section (see Box 16.4), whose function is *to demonstrate and speculate on the meaning and the value of the study.* Many Discussion sections are very highly speculative. If one considers such words as *maybe, perhaps, conceivably, possibly, seems* as markers of speculation, doubt or tentativeness, then the Discussion section of a scientific paper is at least as speculative as a piece of – say – art criticism.

It is this section that offers an opportunity to talk about what the study really means without the constraints of scientific rigour which obtain elsewhere: contrast the use of the word 'significant' (which has a very precise statistical meaning in the Results section) and the use of words such as 'interesting' and so on in this section. Discussions vary greatly in length, and conventions differ from journal to journal: the *BMJ* often has a one-sentence summary of Results at the start of this section, for example, and typically the elements here are (as in the paper quoted) presented in unpredictable order, mixed in with other things.

How does this work in practice? If one puts these sixteen moves together, in the order suggested, the result will be a research article which will be perceived as appropriately written.

The general approach indicated above has been widely used in the teaching of academic reading and writing, and there has been some discussion recently about whether teaching individuals to write up their work like this will help them to think more clearly as well: in other words, whether attention to form can improve the quality of ideas.

Box 16.2 Introduction

1. Ankle injuries are one of the **commonest** causes of referral to accident and emergency departments and

2. account for 2% of all radiographic requests.[1]

3. Discussion of the treatment of patients with ankle injuries during a regular audit meeting of the orthopaedic and accident and emergency departments had **suggested** that treatment could be improved to reduce the proportion of patients who had radiography, to reduce the number of patients without fractures who were referred to the fracture clinics, and to ensure adequate treatment and follow-up of patients with ligamentous injuries of the ankle.

4. We therefore **performed** an audit to confirm that these problems existed and to explore ways of improving treatment.

Packer GJ, Goring CC, Gayner AD and Craxford AD (1991) Audit of Ankle Injuries in an Accident and Emergency Department. *BMJ*. **302**: 885–7.

1. Laparoscopic cholecystectomy is **increasingly accepted** as the treatment of choice in the elective management of symptomatic cholelithiasis.

2. The presence of empyema or severe inflammation of the gallbladder was initially regarded as a contraindication to this technique.[1,2] **Nevertheless**, laparoscopic cholecystectomy for acute cholecystitis has been reported with a degree of technical success in limited series.[3-5]

3. Since the introduction of laparoscopic cholecystectomy we have **attempted** it in all patients presenting with symptomatic gallstones, even when acute inflammation is suspected.

4. We **describe** our initial experience in those patients who presented with empyema or severe acute inflammation of the gallbladder.

Wilson RG, Macintyre IMC, Nixon SJ, Saunders JH, Varma JS and King PM (1992) Laparoscopic Cholecystectomy as a Safe and Effective Treatment for Severe Acute Cholecystitis. *BMJ*. **305**: 394–6.

It seems not impossible that one can create a habit of thinking in this way, but that the two are not inevitably linked is clear from the paper in Box 16.5 , which is offered as a brief – and I hope relatively clear – example of how the system works (the idea of the experiment is taken from a sketch by Spike Milligan).

Box 16.3 Methods
Method

5. **Identify the population**
    (exemplified in every paper)
    and assert inclusiveness (typically with a word like *all, every, each*)
    . . . **all** 77 general practices in the three district health authorities covered by Warwickshire Health Services Authority were invited to participate.

6. **Describe procedures**
    (exemplified in every paper)
    and validate them (by reference to literature, pilot study or consultation procedure)
    . . . a series of postgraduate meetings, or focus groups, was held in all three districts and all 77 practices were invited.

7. **Name statistical/other tests: often linked to justification of choice**
    . . . cost-effectiveness . . . was determined by comparing the costs of feedback with the incidence of reported effects . . . This approach was adopted because observed effects could not accurately be quantified in money terms.[27,28]

Results

8. **Describe adjustments and exclusions (describes numerical disparities between the idealized research design and what actually happened)**
    Of the 77 practices, 52 (68%) . . . were recruited to the study.

9. **Tables**
    (exemplified in every study, although sometimes in a brief and perfunctory manner)

10. **Figures in words**
    (exemplified in every study – a discursive listing of figures, most often as percentages, raw numbers, even expressions of quantity: *many, few* etc.)

11. **Evaluate the findings objectively, usually with reference to statistical significance**
    . . . the 16 smaller practices . . . exhibited significantly higher values for several indicators of preventive practice than the 36 large practices.

(All examples from Szczepura A, Wilmot J, Davies C and Fletcher J (1994) Effectiveness and cost for different strategies for information feedback in general practice. *British Journal of General Practice*. **44**: 19–24)

Box 16.4 Discussion

12. **Validate procedures and findings by reference to comparable studies (this is more common than the other possibility: Contrast findings with those in comparable studies)**

    The use of secondary prophylaxis has not been previously recorded, though unpublished data from the Second International Study of Infarct Survival[13] also found an underuse of beta blockers . . .

    . . . age and sex distribution of the patients was very similar to that previously reported.

13. **Make claim about what the study has shown, demonstrated or suggests**

    This study shows that in the northern region many patients . . . were discharged from hospital receiving suboptimum treatment.

14. **Acknowledge limitations**

    From our data we have no clear idea why treatment was not given . . .

15. **Point the way forward (by recommendations, or statements about what should happen, either in research or practice)**

    . . . we repeat the apparently unheeded advice that beta blockers and aspirin should be given to all patients who can tolerate them.

16. **Evaluate the meaning of the project (state what it suggests is likely to be the case: comment on what is certain or doubtful, on whether findings are satisfactory)**

    . . . pharmacological reasons for not giving treatment may form only part of the picture . . .

(All examples from Eccles M and Bradshaw C (1991) Use of secondary prophylaxis against myocardial infarction in the North of England. *BMJ.* **302**: 91–2)

Box 16.5 The influence of utterances on spreads and contiguous parsnips

J. Skelton (University of Birmingham)

Introduction

1. The ability to persuade people by flattery is a crucial skill in modern life.

2. A number of studies[1,2] have demonstrated a causal connection between success, as measured by the PIE (peers' increased envy) scale[3] and an ability to strike attitudes in a subtly oleaginous manner.

3. No study, however, has demonstrated whether it is possible to achieve effects in the physical world in a controlled manner by the use of language alone.

4. The aim of this study is to provide a partial answer to this question.

Method

5. Fifty men and 50 women were recruited at random from the practice database. Using a professional linguist as consultant, a list of utterances was drawn up suitable for M M, M F, F M, F F dyads (see Appendix).

6. Three tables were then set up in adjoining rooms, in order to minimize variation in environment. On the table in one room (Station A) a parsnip was installed and 2 oz of butter (unsalted) placed at a distance of 3 cm. In a neighbouring room (Station B) margarine was substituted for butter and in a third room (Station C) the parsnip was unaccompanied. In all three rooms a north easterly draught was detected. Dyads were placed at each station in turn, and assigned roles as utterers or listeners. Utterers then recited gender-appropriate language drawn from the list of utterances in the Appendix.

Every instantiation of each utterance was recorded on video. At the end of the investigation the parsnips, butter and margarine were weighed to establish whether transfer of mass had occurred.

7. **Analysis**

An analysis was undertaken, using a form of wishful thinking.

Results

8. One respondent, a male aged 83, was found to be deaf and unable to act as listener, despite a great deal of shouting. His results were excluded from the final analysis. One female participant spoke only Hungarian. Consideration was given to obtaining a consignment of Hungarian parsnips, but this suggestion was rejected. Her utterances were relayed to listeners and parsnips through an interpreter. This left a total of 97 participants (M = 48; F = 49).

9. There was a high degree of uniformity for parsnip and spread mass before and after intervention. At Station A, which had the largest parsnip mass, the overall change was of the same order of magnitude as at Station B.

10. The results are shown in Table 1.

Table 1 Net weights (in grams) before and after experimental treatment

	Station A		Station B		Station C	
	Before	After	Before	After	Before	After
Parsnip	422	422	240	240	357	357
Spread	100	100	100	100	—	—

11. There was no significant difference between the parsnip masses before and after intervention.

Discussion

12. The findings were in accord with views expressed elsewhere.[4]

13. The study demonstrates that fine words butter no parsnips. Language on its own was unable to transfer mass to parsnips either from contiguous spreads (Stations A and B) or from a distance (Station C).

14. The presence of the slight wind, however, was an unexpected variable, and results should be viewed with caution.

15. The similar pattern of results at Stations A and B leaves open the possibility that parsnips are perhaps unable to tell margarine from butter, and this hypothesis should be tested.

Appendix

A selection of phrases used in dyads:

M M
1. I wish I earned half your salary
2. Have you ever thought of turning professional?
3. What's your secret with women?

M F
1. You're 40! You're having me on!
2. You're so much cleverer than me
3. Of course I'm listening to you

F F
1. I know *I* couldn't cope with a job and a family
2. It must be wonderful, being a size 10
3. That man's looking at you

F M
1. Older men have such maturity
2. You must spend *ages* working out
3. Darling, it's enormous

References

1. Skelton J (1996) 'If only people were nicer to me.' *British Journal for the Bewildered.* **22**: 101–2.

2. Lizard L (1994) What to say to the opposite sex with smouldering glances. *Journal of Doctor–Nurse Romances.* **18**: 123.

3. Zygote W and Aardvark A (1992) Principles for deciding who should be named as first author: measuring success in a university. *British Journal of Professional Pique.* **27**: 8–9.

4. The little old lady at number 32 (personal communication)

QUESTIONS AND ANSWERS

- **What matters most, my science or my style?** For quantitative studies, bad style can usually be rescued at editorial level in a way that bad science cannot be. For qualitative studies, particularly those which are very ethnographic in orientation, it is a little harder to separate the ideas from the words that express them. In general, however, the main reason for developing good style is to clarify good ideas.

- **Which journals are worth publishing in?** One way of measuring this is by citation rates: how often do people in other journals make reference to the journal? However, it depends on your priority: a middlebrow, popular journal with wide readership (original studies published in the *BMJ* have a wide circulation, which may be a different matter) may be an effective way to change practice, for example, even if it does not carry much academic weight.

- **When should I start considering where to get my work published?** You should be thinking about this from the outset, and certainly before you begin writing you should have a very clear idea of your audience and the conventions associated with that journal. Do not start writing until you have read your targeted journal's 'Notes to contributors'.

- **How easy is it to get published?** The top journals are very difficult, even for experienced researchers, but not impossible. Any reasonable study will find a home somewhere reasonable, and to be frank, most semi-reasonable things can be placed somewhere. Do not be disheartened by rejection: take seriously the reviewers' comments which you will be sent by refereed journals, and if you end up submitting the same piece to several places, have the patience to learn the different conventions demanded by the different house styles. Of course, it can all be a bit of a lottery: a former colleague of mine was once told her paper was fine but too short by one reviewer, fine but too long by another. On the whole, however, reviewers give detailed and useful help, and will often provide real insight into your work.

- **Should I get anyone to read my work before I send it off?** Yes, if at all possible – if nothing else, a colleague or friend will be able to point out that the things you have not bothered explaining because familiarity has made them seem obvious to you are, in fact, incomprehensible to others. Note, however, that most people can be easily hurt by negative criticism of their studies: choose carefully (and if a friend asks you to perform the same service, do so with tact).

Further reading

There is no shortage, in medicine, of books about how to write. Two which are well known are:

Huth E (1990) *How to Write and Publish Papers in the Medical Sciences*. Williams and Wilkins, Baltimore.

Cormack D (1994) *Writing for Health Care Professions*. Blackwell, Oxford.

Some conventions are set out in the following, although they are followed to varying degrees by different journals. Generally, the more highbrow or more quantitative the journal, the more rigorously it will be in accord with these precepts.

International Committee of Medical Journal Editors (1991) Uniform Requirements for Manuscripts Submitted to Biomedical Journals. *BMJ.* **302**: 338–41.

There is a more detailed analysis of the genre of academic medicine in:

Skelton J (1994) Analysis of the Structure of Original Research Papers: an Aid to Writing Original Papers for Publication. *British Journal of General Practice.* **44**: 455–9.

Other texts mentioned are:

Bartlett FC (1932) *Remembering.* Cambridge University Press, Cambridge.

Gilbert GN and Mulkay M (1984) *Opening Pandora's Box: a Sociological Analysis of Scientific Discourse.* Cambridge University Press, Cambridge.

Goodman KS and Fleming JT (eds) (1969) *Psycholinguistics and the Teaching of Reading.* International Reading Association, Newark, Delaware.

Swales JM (1990) *Genre Analysis: English in Academic and Research Settings.* Cambridge University Press, Cambridge.

Aladdin and the enchanted lamp, in *Tales From the Thousand and One Nights* (tr. NJ Dawood). Penguin, Harmondsworth: 1954, 1986.

Index